Heartwarming Short Stories for Seniors - Golden Pages of Ageless Tales

Large Print Book for Seniors with True Stories that Inspire, Stimulate the Mind and Ward Off Dementia

Grace Ellington

Contents

A Kiss on the Water Tower

I stepped off the train and felt the warmth of my hometown surrounding me. The air was filled with the scent of freshly cut grass, and the sound of crickets hummed in my ears. After a year spent on the East Coast attending an Ivy League school, I had forgotten how comforting it was to return to a place with such strong roots.

My sister Elaine greeted me with a large smile as she picked me up from the station. "Welcome home!" she exclaimed, hugging me tightly.

I laughed and hugged her back, relieved she was genuinely excited to see me. After being away for so long, I guess I let myself believe I wouldn't be welcome anymore. "How's everyone?" I asked.

Elaine filled me in on the latest happenings while I was away. She told me about the new Italian restaurant, the high school's surprising basketball victory at the league championships, and the record-breaking amount of money raised at the Sunday church bake sale. I listened attentively, marveling at how little my hometown had changed during my absence.

When we arrived home, our parents were waiting to greet me. They hugged me and then immediately launched into a discussion about the family business. "You should come work with me," my father said.

"We can get you started right after graduation," my mother chimed in.

I nodded, trying to avoid disappointing them, but I knew in my heart that working in the family business wasn't what I wanted. I didn't want to run a little hardware store. I didn't go to school for that and I could have just gone to community college to learn what I needed to learn to do it. Actually, I didn't really have to go to college at all to help there. I'd been working there my entire childhood.

Over the next few days, I attempted to reconnect with old childhood friends. However, everyone seemed to have moved on without me.

Whenever I mentioned college or my experiences on the East Coast, it seemed they listened politely but with no interest at all. I felt like a stranger. I guess I wasn't the same either.

One day, while browsing the local bookstore, I met Rose. She was studying to become a teacher and had a passion for literature. Our conversation flowed effortlessly, and we bonded over our shared love for the written word. Over the following weeks, we spent all of our free time together, exploring the town and reliving our shared experiences. I think if she wasn't a few years older than me almost done with her post graduate work, we might have been romantic.

As time passed, my father wanted a commitment from me.

"We've invested so much time and money into your education."

"It's time for you to start thinking about your future."

"You can't just live life willy-nilly, boy. You need to make a decision."

I couldn't argue with my father's logic, but I also couldn't bear the thought of living life without any sense of freedom or independence. The more I pondered, the more certain I became I didn't want to work in the family business. I wasn't even sure I wanted to settle down and start a family after college was over. I didn't know if I ever would. I still had dreams of experiencing life beyond my hometown or the college campus.

I confided in Rose about my conflicting desires and provided me with some much-needed perspective. "You don't have to choose between your family and your dreams," she said, "but they need to choose whether or not they'll support you.

She shared stories from her own experiences growing up in a small town in California, where she felt suffocated with the pressure to conform to her community's expectations. She was supposed to marry the football quarterback and be a housewife.

They'd been sweethearts forever and this idea she should have her own career wasn't really common back in the early seventies.

It wasn't until Rose moved across the country to attend college that she found her independence and learned to follow her passions. She followed her dreams and her family was angry but the anger passed and soon her family was supportive. Seeing the strength that Rose possessed and how she lived her life on her own terms, I began to question my own values and desires. I started to see that following my passion for literature and education was just as important as fulfilling my familial obligations.

On our final night together, Rose had a surprise for me. We climbed to the top of the water tower, a spot nobody had visited for years since the old steel tower had been converted into a modern water storage tank. As I gazed out at the vast expanse of land around me, I was struck by the sheer beauty of my hometown.

"I'm happy I met you," I said to Rose. "I believe you've saved me from losing sight of what I want in life."

Rose smiled at me, knowing I was finally starting to appreciate the value of my aspirations. We held hands as we watched the bright orange sun set below the horizon. Even though we knew our time together would soon end, we cherished the moments we shared and recognized their significance. We shared a kiss that night. It would turn out to be the only kiss the two of us ever shared.

The next day, as I boarded the train to the East Coast, I felt a mix of sadness and excitement. For the first time in my life, I knew what I wanted and what I was willing to fight for: my independence and the pursuit of my passions. Even though it meant disappointing my parents and leaving behind the hometown that I had grown up dutifully bound to, I realized that it was time to stop playing it safe and finally take charge of my life.

As the train pulled away from the station, I turned to wave goodbye to Rose as she disappeared among the crowd.

I knew that I would always remember the lessons she had taught me and the memories we shared. And, of course, I would always remember that kiss on the water tower.

Years later, I retired from a thirty-five-year career as a professor. My cousin Charlie ended up taking over the hardware store and he came alone with Elaine and my mother to my retirement dinner. Dad passed away a few years back but he and I made our peace about my career twenty years before he died. I invited Rose but she couldn't make it because it coincided with her daughter's college graduation. She sent me a card, and that seemed appropriate since we stayed in touch over the years but only with Christmas cards and birthday wishes.

I'll admit to a lot of idle daydreaming over the years about how life might have gone if that kiss on the water tower had been only one of many. I never regretted leaving it at one kiss, though, not any more than I regretted that one kiss in the first place. I had the career I chose and I had the wife and children I chose as well. In many ways, I have Rose to thank for all of it. Since her advice was to forge my own path, though, I suppose I ought to thank myself.

Fire Boy

I had always dreamed of seeing the world beyond my small hometown in Iowa. And when I saw the recruiters at my high school telling stories of adventure and valor, I was hooked. I signed up right then and there, not quite old enough to vote but ready to serve my country. I proposed to my girlfriend but she said she couldn't get engaged and then wonder if I would even come home.

By the time I arrived in Vietnam, I had heard all sorts of horror stories about the war. The stories were overblown and crazy but nothing could have prepared me for the reality I saw when I arrived. The heat and humidity were stifling, and the constant sound of gunfire and explosions was overwhelming. I couldn't believe this was my adventure.

I was stuck there, though. I had to adapt and since everyone there had to adapt, it was easy to find ways to do it. I fell into a routine of daily patrols and strategic strikes, working alongside my fellow soldiers to accomplish our mission. The truth was most of the time there was sheer boredom. It was drudgery except for moments of overpowering intensity.

We were told constantly that we were comrades in arms; we were family. Eventually, we all felt that way. We watched each other's backs, shared our rations and joked around to keep our spirits up. One of the soldiers in my platoon and I quickly became close friends. Jack was a couple of years older than me, with deep set brown eyes, a square jaw, and a contagious grin that could light up a dark jungle trail. Jack grew up on a farm in Michigan and was drafted while he was working as a mechanic.

He always had a way of calming me down whenever I got worked up about something. He was like a big brother, I guess. While we were out on patrol one day, Jack pulled me aside. "Hey" he said, putting his hand on my shoulder. "You calm down because you're going to be fine. You have fire inside you, brother. Don't lose it."

Fire inside of me. He said those words just as I was feeling a bit like a coward. I was taken aback. Jack somehow knew exactly when to say what needed to be said. His words lingered with me long after he said them. As time passed, we continued on with our patrols, securing areas, searching tunnels and making life hard for the NVA, an enemy we never really saw up close and never knew as more than just the people trying to kill us, when we could. We marched in the heat, battled the elements, and tried to stay alive. Nights were filled with exhaustion, injury, and occasional respite if we were lucky.

For me, the hardest moment of the war came during one of our most dangerous missions. Our company had received intel that the NVA were stockpiling weapons and ammunition deep in a jungle stronghold, which made it a high-priority target. It was risky but necessary. Our superiors knew it would be dangerous, so they sent in three platoons to increase our chances of success.

As soon as we arrived at the location, we realized just how well-armed the enemy was. They started shooting as soon as we got within range, and soon the trees around us were exploding with gunfire. We took cover behind whatever we could find and returned fire where possible.

During the chaos, I heard Jack shouting out to me. "Hey, Fire Boy!" he yelled. "Stop staring and start shooting!"

Despite the danger, I couldn't help but laugh. Jack always had a way of brightening up even the darkest moments. I looked over and saw him grinning at me through the smoke and gunfire, his eyes alight with fierce determination. We fought hard for what felt like hours, taking out enemy soldiers one by one. But then, I heard a strangled gasp from somewhere in the trees. I turned around and saw Jack falling to the ground, blood staining his shirt.

I rushed to his side and saw that he had been shot in the chest. He was still breathing, but it was shallow and labored. Tears streamed down my face as he looked up at me. "Tell my wife...tell her I love her," he gasped.

I nodded but said, "You're going to tell her. You're gonna make it, Jack!"

I knew that it was a lie and Jack knew it, too. "Come on, Fire Boy," he started but his eyes started to glaze over as the light left his body. He was gone. The rest of the mission became a blur. I didn't even remember firing my weapon; all I could think about was Jack. My best friend in Vietnam was gone, and I would never forget him.

When the fire was over, I carried Jack back to base. I wouldn't let anyone help. We held a memorial service there. His wife and family weren't there, of course, and I knew they'd have their own memorial service when he returned to them.

I wrote letters to his wife and told him how his last words were to make sure to tell her that he loved her. It wasn't exactly true. His last words were, "Come on, Fire Boy." The little lie never weighed on my conscience.

Over the months to come, I realized the profound impact he had had on me. His admonition not to lose the fire inside stayed with me. The way Jack showed me how to stay positive and hopeful even in the darkest moments, and it was something that I knew I would always carry with me.

After Jack's death, everything changed. I began to see the war through different eyes. It wasn't just about fighting for my country; it was about making sure that no more soldiers had to die the way Jack did. It was a sense of purpose that drove me forward. Officially, soldiers weren't allowed to write on their helmets but everyone did. They wrote things like War is Good Business and plenty of punchlines to dirty jokes. I used a permanent marker to write Fire Boy in big block letters.

I found myself working harder than ever before, volunteering for extra missions and taking on additional responsibilities.

I knew that I was doing everything I could to make a difference. And while it didn't bring Jack back, it gave me some solace to know that I was fighting for a cause that was larger than myself. It wasn't about winning the war. It wasn't about politics. It was Jack dying in my arms and Fire Boy making sure nobody on any mission ever looked up at him to tell him something to say to his wife back home.

When I finally returned home from Vietnam, I almost reenlisted the very next day. There were more Jack's I wanted to keep from dying. Fire Boy's work wasn't done. My father convinced me to spend at least a few months home first. I did and this time before I reenlisted, my girlfriend not only accepted my proposal but we married.

I didn't return to Vietnam. The army promoted me for valor in combat and sent me to officers training school. By the time I was done, the war was over. I spent another twenty-two years in the Army and never fought overseas again. Looking back now, it's hard to believe that so much time has passed since those days in Vietnam. But the lessons that I learned there have stayed with me, shaping who I am today. I miss Jack every day and to this day, everyone still calls me Fire Boy.

Rachel's Necklace

I know people say things like this all the time but I remember the summer of 1985 like it was yesterday. It was sunny but not too hot and in my little town in the Midwest, that meant one thing. It meant I had to go outside and play. For me, that meant running to my best friend's house. Rachel lived two houses down but one block behind my house.

Since the weather was perfect, I already knew what we were going to do. We tried to do this particular thing every time we possibly could. We were going fishing because girls were just as good at catching fish as boys. The only problem was, neither of us had ever caught a big fish.

We both lived in the heart of the Midwest, surrounded by vast cornfields and lazy rivers that ran through them. To get to the river where we planned to catch our first big fish, we would have to ride our bicycles somehow managing to carry our fishing rods, bait, and a tackle box. We usually fished a closer river but this day we really wanted a big fish so we pedaled with all our gear to a new spot we'd heard about from our older brothers.

We arrived at the river where an old wooden bridge connected both sides. The water flowed slowly, and we could see algae growing on some rocks. It was peaceful, with birds tweeting, butterflies flitting around, and the rustling of the trees. Rachel spotted a snake slithering into the bushes and shrieked, but I assured her that it wouldn't bother us. We found a suitable area near the riverbank, laid out a blanket we had packed, and began our quest to catch fish.

We cast lines without success, waiting for over an hour, using mixed baits. I always baited Rachel's hook for her because she got squeamish and I didn't. With no success, boredom set in, and Rachel suggested we take a swim in the river to cool off. At first, I refused, scared that I might drown, but she insisted it would be safe.

Reluctantly, I agreed, and after finding an area, we jumped into the water. Rachel swam like a pro while I half-floated, half-swam around with my head barely above the water. She was like a mermaid and I was more like a princess taking a bath.

We forgot about fishing for a while and I thought about how swimming wasn't all that scary. By the time we got out, I was already much better and even went underneath the surface a few times and tried to swim more like Rachel. We laughed and smiled and then got back to our quest.

Girls were just as good at fishing as boys!

We said that a few times as we climbed back onto the bank and made our way to our blanket by the bridge. As we headed back to the spot our fishing gear lay, though. Rachel noticed her necklace was missing. It was a gift from her grandfather on her seventh birthday and for almost four years, she wore it every day. Rachel sat down and started to cry. I sat next to her and tried to reassure her.

"Don't worry! We'll find it in no time at all." Of course, I had no idea how we would find it in no time at all. I just said that because my best friend was crying.

We searched for hours and had no luck at all. Two very sad girls went home that afternoon, I can tell you.

We hadn't caught a big fish and she'd lost something very important to her.

Kids are resilient, though, and so were we. The next day, we returned to the spot just to search for the necklace. We didn't find it, of course, but we spent three or four pleasant hours swimming while we searched. That went on for a few days and then my brother teased us about not catching fish so the next day we brought the fishing poles again.

Every day except for Sunday, we went to that spot. We went and we always spent the first hour or so searching for the necklace and, of course, never finding it. We also never caught a big fish. We caught some bluegill and a few small trout but nothing big enough to show off to our brothers. By the time the middle of August rolled around, Rachel and I were closer than ever. The summer was magical and there were only a few more weeks before we would both start our new adventure, junior high.

Our brothers terrorized us with stories about how hard schoolwork was in junior high school and it motivated us even more. We went to our fishing hole with even more determination those last two weeks. We brought worms and crickets and even put bells on the ends of the poles so we wouldn't miss out on any bites. For those two weeks, we didn't even search for the necklace.

We remained bright and optimistic all the way through those two weeks but I have to admit that we didn't bike very fast on our last day. We felt desperate but the optimism was gone. Maybe there wasn't even the slightest amount of hope. There was plenty of desperation and Rachel even put her worm on her hook all by herself.

The hours passed and we were ready to pack it in. Since we had just one nightcrawler left, though, I put it on a hook and cast one last time. It plopped into the river and Rachel said, "I don't care how hard seventh grade is; we're going to be best friends forever."

I didn't get a chance to agree with her because my pole jerked hard!

It was a big fish! It was a really big fish. I held onto the pole and we watched it bend like it would snap in two. I should tell you that even though we thought girls were just as good as boys at fishing, neither of us really knew what to do at all. I thought the fish would pull me right into the river. Rachel came up behind me and wrapped her arms around my waist. She pulled me backward while I did my best to reel the fish in.

Keep the tip up.

That was the advice my father gave me when he taught me to fish so that's what I did. I kept the tip up and I reeled and Rachel held onto me. I think it probably took about five minutes to get that fish onto the riverbank but Rachel and I thought it was a battle of epic proportions, like an ancient castle siege. The fish was a big channel cat, and it seemed to me to be the biggest fish anyone ever caught in all of history.

It was actually about ten pounds, not even close to a state record. We found that out when we got home, breathless and tired, two girls covered with river mud and holding up the fish like it was some kind of treasure.

It was.

My mother took pictures of the two of us holding the fish and my brother stared enviously. My mother called Rachel's mother and invited her parents and her brother over because there was more than enough for everyone.

It was the perfect end to the perfect summer.

But there was more!

You'll never believe what we found in that catfish's stomach.

Well, I imagine you've guessed. When Daddy gutted it, something glittered and Rachel cried out, "My necklace!" Sure enough, it was there and no worse for the wear. She wore it that night as we ended the summer with fried catfish, potato salad, and pecan pie.

Junior high wasn't nearly as hard as our brothers told us it would be, of course, but it brought changes. Rachel and I remained fast friends but going fishing didn't seem as fun to us as going to dances or hanging out at the arcade in the hopes of seeing this boy or that boy we liked. We were fast friends in high school, too, but by then the boys commanded most of our time and most of our attention.

She went to college and I went to a different college and these days we only see each other on Thanksgiving, Christmas, and Easter because we always bring our families home to spend those holidays with our parents. Sometimes, we'll take our kids to our favorite fishing spot. Sometimes we don't. I'll tell you one thing that happens every time I see her. She wears her necklace.

Summers with Nana

I wasn't thrilled about spending my summer caring for my Nana, but I didn't complain. I knew she needed my help and since my older brother was already in college, the job fell to me. So, I begrudgingly packed my bags and headed to her house in the countryside. I was seventeen years old and there were a lot of things I would have liked better than a summer with my ailing grandmother but in my family, you didn't argue about things like this.

Pulling up to her house, I was struck with a wave of nostalgia. I spent many summers here as a young child, running through fields and playing in the stream nearby. But now, things were different, and I felt like I had outgrown it all. I wasn't going to marvel at daisies or stare in wonder at cottontail rabbits. As I walked to the house, I saw Nana's flowerbeds, once carefully managed, were overgrown now. Her garden gnomes which I had found so cute and wonderful seemed sad and lonely guardians of a dying house.

I stepped inside the house, and Nana greeted me with a hug. Her frail frame seemed even smaller than I remembered, and her once sharp mind was now forgetful. It made me sad. I was seventeen, though. I wasn't used to feeling sad for real reasons. I wasn't lost in the temporary sadness of an argument with a boyfriend or a concert I couldn't attend. This was real sadness, and I wanted to run away. I couldn't help feeling guilty for wishing I could be anywhere else.

The days went by slowly. I took care of Nana's needs and tried to fill the silence. I found myself longing for the sound of my friends' laughter, the buzz of people around me, and the freedom of being young and carefree. I even missed some of the girls with haughty dispositions and mean attitudes. I began hiding away in my room, scrolling through magazines or staring blankly out of the window. Anything to pass the time until I could leave.

I couldn't leave fast enough when the summer ended. I was ready before the sun came up. I made Nana breakfast and after she ate, I gave her a hug. My aunt and Uncle would be here during the school year. When the hug finished, she said, "I'll miss you Jaybird."

She hadn't called me Jaybird since I was seven or eight years old.

I thought about that for many weeks. Every time a teacher called out my name for roll call, I imagined she said, Jaybird Tucker instead of Jayne Tucker. I couldn't understand it because all of my memories of the summer were unhappy but I missed Nana. Of course, by the time the next summer rolled around and I was once again instructed to go to her, I wasn't happy at all. I was eighteen but since my father was paying for my college, I felt trapped.

Or maybe I just wanted to go but didn't want to admit it to myself.

That summer was different. The very first morning, while fetching ingredients from the pantry for breakfast, I overheard Nana talking to her old photo album. At first, I thought it was her forgetfulness talking, but then I noticed that she was telling stories. Stories about her childhood, her family, and her adventures. I was fascinated by her tales, and soon, I found myself asking questions and listening to her intently.

Nana's stories took me on a journey through her life, and I was enthralled. One of her most hilarious tales was of her attempting to ride her pet goat when she was little, only to fall off and land on a cactus. Even at her age, her sense of humor hadn't faltered, and we laughed together as she retold the story.

As the summer progressed, I realized how much I had misjudged my time with Nana. I may have come here to help care for her, but she, too, had cared for me. I started to see the beauty in being present, living each moment to its fullest, and cherishing memories. I didn't want to leave when the summer ended but college beckoned. Unlike the first summer, I lingered on the last day and didn't drive away until Nana was asleep.

That third summer was different. I knew from the moment I stepped through the door and Nana couldn't even get up to greet me that she didn't have much time. Although it was bittersweet, I cherished every moment. Nana and I reminisced about our past summers; we played games, baked our favorite treats, and talked for hours. We even went to the stream where we used to play when I was little, and I saw a different side of my Nana. She sang old folk songs that she had learned from her mother, and I felt like I was experiencing a part of history.

It wasn't until that summer that I realized that all the time I had spent with Nana over the two prior summers produced the happiest memories I had. As the days passed, I could tell that Nana was growing weaker, and it broke my heart. The last day before I left, I told her how much I loved her and how much I appreciated my time with her. She said I was her Jaybird and I filled her with my songs. I think I cried the whole way as I drove home.

As winter approached that year, I received news that Nana had passed away. My mother called me in the morning about an hour before my last semester final exam. I felt numb as I took the exam and then numb as I drove home. As the preacher spoke, I felt like most of the people at the service didn't know Nana like I did. I felt like they couldn't possibly be as sad and unhappy about her passing as I was. I felt like I hurt more because I loved Nana more than anyone else. I guess a lot of people feel that way when someone important to them passes away.

Of course, it didn't take long for me to realize someone else loving Nana didn't take away from what I had with her. That summer may have been the last one, but it was the most transformative one for me. I learned that sometimes the greatest moments in life are the simple ones. The time spent with loved ones is priceless, and if anything, my time with Nana made me realize the value of slowing down and enjoying life's little moments.

Nana's stories, values, and lessons stayed with me long after she was gone. In fact, they stay with me still. Looking back, I'm grateful for those summers and often laugh at the younger me who didn't want to spend them with her.

Every summer, I visit her to arrange the flowers and the garden gnomes on her grave. When I do, I can't help but smile at all the happy memories we shared. I always feel like she's looking down on me, proud of the person I have become. I always thank her when I'm there. I have a great deal to be thankful for because Nana gave me a wonderful gift. She gave me a gift that no one can ever take away, and that was the understanding of empathy, compassion, and time well-spent.

The Popular Girl

I used to hang out with Alex all the time when we were little. We would do everything together and always have each other's backs. But as we entered high school, things started to change. Alex became more outgoing and popular while I remained my quiet and reserved self. I watched from the sidelines as Alex made new friends and became more involved in different activities. Meanwhile, I felt like I was being left behind.

I guess we also both paid closer attention to the fact that I was boy and she was a girl. It never seemed to matter in elementary school and junior high. We were friends. She was my first kiss just because we both wanted to know what a kiss was like. We were eleven years old when that happened and there was no romance involved at all. Our friendship continued as though nothing happened. In high school, though, there was a different kind of outlook, like it wasn't possible for boys and girls to be friends but always romantic interests and crushes.

All of that didn't matter to me because I'd never much cared what my peers thought of me. I kept to myself most of the time and so I never felt like there was anything to lose by not impressing others. Of course, the exception was Alex and when she left me behind, it hurt. I resented Alex for that but I didn't know how to communicate my feelings to her. Instead, I just kept quiet and pretended like everything was okay, even though it wasn't.

One day at school, I snapped at her. She asked how I was doing and I replied with, "What do you care? Go ask all your new friends how they're doing." I felt immediately horrible about and I hurried away. The look of hurt and surprise on her face when I snapped at her didn't leave my mind for the rest of the day. It was still in my mind in the morning, too.

That day, Alex invited me to a party at her house. I accepted, just happy she wasn't angry with me about snapping at her.

I was also excited to see her and hang out with her. The party was two days later and I felt happy and cheerful as those two days passed.

But when I got there, I felt like an outsider. Everyone was talking and laughing, and I struggled to keep up with their conversations. As the night went on, Alex seemed to be having a great time with all her friends while I sat on the couch by myself. I tried to join in on the fun, but I felt like I was just getting in the way. Eventually, I couldn't take it anymore and just left without saying goodbye to anyone. Alex tried calling me but whenever my parents told me it was her, I came up with an excuse not to go to the phone. The party was on Friday night. I ignored six or seven calls from her on Saturday.

I still felt angry and hurt on Sunday. When the phone rang on Sunday morning, I was alone in the house. I listened and stared. I didn't want to answer but since my parents weren't home, I thought it might be them. I answered, afraid it might be Alex calling. It wasn't Alex.

It was Willie French's mother. He'd been in a car accident and he was in the hospital. She thought maybe a visit would cheer him up. I'd grown up with him. We didn't have a friendship as close as my friendship with Alex but if you told me to write down five friends, I would only be able to come up with two, Alex and Willie.

I got on my bike and pedaled like a madman. When I arrived at the hospital, I saw Alex getting out of her mother's car. We both looked at each other and then looked away. She had an arrangement of flowers and I realized she was there to see Willie, too.

We didn't talk until we walked past the hospital gift shop and went inside. Then, we awkwardly discussed what I should get for Willie. We settled on a handheld electronic game. I was there to visit Willie but it seemed like Alex was the entire focus of all my thoughts. I felt a little guilty about that.

The visit with Willie was really difficult. He was really beat up.

We kept a brave face and laughed and joked but by the time we left, we were both overwhelmed. We walked to the front of the hospital and that was when Alex said, "I'm sorry about the party. I didn't mean to make you feel left out."

It was a peace offering but I replied bitterly. "It's not just about the party. It's about everything. You've changed so much since we were kids, and I'm still the same. I just... you used to care about doing things with me. Now you don't. You're the most popular girl in school and I'm still me."

"I know I've been busy with other things, but that doesn't mean I stopped caring about you," Alex said, "and you're wrong. You have changed. You don't understand, James. I can't be your friend anymore."

That shocked me. It shocked me right out of the bitterness and brought me right back to a desperate sense of loss. "Why not?" I whispered.

I saw her cheeks color. It seemed strange for her to blush at a time like this. She finally said, "Because you've changed."

And then she kissed me.

It was our second kiss, five and a half years after our first kiss... but it was the first one, too.

When we looked at each other afterward, she said, "I *have* been avoiding you. I *have* been hiding. I was afraid of what just happened, afraid that we would stop being friends because... because I want more. I was afraid I would lose my best friend and I wouldn't get to be more than friends, either."

I didn't have any idea what to say.

I had a pretty good idea what to do, though, and I kissed her.

Of course, nobody was surprised that we were suddenly together. It didn't surprise me that our parents reacted by saying, "Of course, you're together," and with similar comments.

What surprised me was that everyone at school seemed to expect it as well. I guess that just goes to show that people see you better than see yourself sometimes.

Five months before my seventeenth birthday, Alex and I stopped being best friends and started being a couple. I guess that's the fondest memory of my life, that moment when things changed there. Of course, there are many other fond memories, like our latest kiss. I guess that's number two or three hundred thousand.

Rusty

I was thirteen years old when my dog died and my first thought was that it might give me enough sympathy that Erica would agree to go to the homecoming dance with me. I know that sounds terrible but I guess it makes it clear just how wrapped up in Erica I felt back then. It was the early 1960s, and I was growing up in a small midwestern town. My parents were both teachers, and my older brother was away at college. Most of the time, it was just me and my dog, Rusty, the scrappy terrier who had been my constant companion since I was five.

Rusty had been sick for a few weeks, but I didn't think much of it. He was always getting into something or other, and we'd taken him to the vet before for one ailment or another. But this time, it was different. Rusty was listless and barely ate, and I knew something was really wrong.

Dad took him to the vet on a Friday afternoon, and when he came back, he looked solemn. "Rusty's not going to make it," he said quietly. "The vet says it's best to put him down now rather than see him suffer."

I was devastated. Rusty had been my constant source of comfort and joy for as long as I could remember. I couldn't bear the thought of life without him. But then, as we were burying Rusty in the backyard and tears streaming down my face, I had a thought. If Erica saw how upset I was about Rusty, maybe she'd feel sorry for me enough to go to the homecoming dance with me.

Yeah, I actually let that thought take hold.

Erica was the prettiest girl in school, blonde and popular, and I'd had a crush on her for as long as I could remember. But she never paid much attention to me. Maybe, just maybe, this could be my chance! The next day at school, if I made sure to cry a little extra during lunch, hoping Erica would notice. "Oh, I'm so sorry about your dog," she would say, putting a hand on my shoulder or even hugging me.

Well, of course, I immediately dismissed the whole fantasy and I felt really bad about it. In fact, I felt guilty enough that at school, I could barely look at her and whenever I did, I ended up feeling very guilty and very sad for Rusty again. After about a week of this, she noticed and came up and said, "What's wrong, Tony?"

Don't ask me how the words came out. I asked, "Do you want to go to the homecoming dance with me?"

My heart skipped a beat. I couldn't believe I said that. It was the exact opposite of what my friends said I was supposed to do. I just blurted the question without even bothering to play it cool.

But a miracle happened. Erica said, "Sure. That will be nice." She smiled brightly and I just stared at her in shock. She asked, "Were you sad because you thought I would say no?"

I shook my head. "Well, I never thought a girl as perfect as you would say yes but..." She blushed a beautiful shade of pink at the compliment and it took me a second to remember to finish. "I was sad because my dog died."

"Oh!" she said and even though she said the word sympathetically, it seemed to me her voice was music. She stepped closer and gave me a hug and it felt to me like that hug lasted forever. It was such a beautiful turn of events. I somehow ended up with a date with Erica without any of the planned manipulation, thoughts of which had me feeling terribly guilty.

From then on, life felt different. With Erica as my date, everything seemed exciting. I mean everything! Geometry was suddenly interesting. Lunch in the cafeteria was suddenly gourmet. As the homecoming dance approached, I could feel a mixture of excitement and nervousness. I'd never been on a real date before, and I wasn't sure what to expect.

When I arrived at Erica's house, corsage in hand and my father's car parked on the street, she looked even more beautiful than ever.

She wore a yellow dress that matched her hair and carried a small purse. I felt my stomach flip with nerves as I greeted her.

"Hi," I said, my voice sounding shaky.

"Hey there," she said, smiling warmly. "Ready to go?"

I nodded, my heart racing as we walked to my car. We chatted nervously on the way to the dance, discussing the latest songs on the radio and the upcoming basketball season. When we got to the high school gym, it was buzzing with excitement. Couples were twirling around the dance floor, enjoying the music and the company of their dates.

Erica and I found a spot at a table near the edge of the room. We talked and laughed, enjoying the novelty of being there together. When a slow song came on, I nervously asked Erica if she wanted to dance. To my surprise, she wanted to. We swayed together in the dim light of the gym, my palms sweaty and my heartbeat pounding in my ears. For a few moments, it felt like time stood still. We didn't sit down again. We danced to the slow songs and the fast songs. We danced to all the songs in between.

After the dance, I drove her home and while we sat in the car parked in front of her house, she said she had a great time.

I blurted out, "best night of my life."

She giggled and said, "me, too." Then, she leaned over and kissed me. It was my first real kiss and if I thought the first dance stopped time for a while, this kiss stopped the world until only the two of us existed.

The next day, she moved to Australia.

I had no idea her father took a job there. I had no idea she was going. She didn't just leave. She stopped by my house to kiss me goodbye and told me the dance with me was her best memory and she would never forget it.

Well, of course I was devastated. It took a long time for the sharp sadness to dull. As time passed, though, my feelings for Erica joined feelings for a number of other crushes that burn so fiercely when we're young.

She wrote to me a few times that first year and I wrote back to her. Gradually, though, we just settled into our separate lives. I had other homecoming dances and she did as well.

Almost forty years have passed since that homecoming dance. I had two dogs who lived long, happy dog lives before passing and their loss hurt me just as much as Rusty's but memories of them outlived them. I have a feeling Rex, my Australian shepherd, is going to outlive me. If not, memories of him will be mine because memories outlive all of us. I guess that homecoming dance and that first kiss are still among my best memories even though I found real love a few years later, love that went beyond the excitement and wonder of youth.

Fitting In

I had always lived in a small town where everyone knew everyone else's business. It was the kind of place where news spread like wildfire and everyone was quick to form an opinion. As a young man, I had big dreams for myself. I wanted to go to college, find a good job and maybe even start a family. But all those dreams came to a screeching halt when I received my draft notice in the mail.

It was 1968, and the Vietnam War was at its peak. At first, I couldn't believe it. I had never thought of myself as a soldier. I was a skinny kid who had never been in a fight in my life. And yet, here I was, being told that I had to leave everything behind and fight in a war I wasn't sure I believed in.

As I prepared to leave for boot camp, I began to feel increasingly isolated. Many of my friends and treated me as a pariah for not protesting the war. They would whisper behind my back, calling me a coward and a traitor. They wanted me to go to Canada. Even people who didn't have a moral objection weren't happy. My parents couldn't hide their disappointment when they saw the draft notice. Of course, they were worried. Still, it meant the time we had together was strained. The same thing happened with my friends who weren't opposed to the war.

I tried to put on a brave face and act as if I was excited about going to war, but deep down, I was terrified. I knew that I would be surrounded by other young men my age, but I wasn't sure if I would be able to make any real friends. It seemed like everyone I met was either angry or scared, and I didn't feel like I fit in with either group.

When I arrived at boot camp, I quickly realized that I was in for a tough ride. The drill sergeants were relentless, barking orders at us recruits all day long.

I found myself struggling to keep up, both physically and emotionally. I felt like I was constantly being pushed to my breaking point, and I didn't know how much more I could take.

As the weeks went by, I began to develop a routine. I would wake up early, complete my morning exercises and then spend the rest of the day drilling and practicing with my fellow recruits. The only time I had to myself was at night when I would lie in bed and think about my family and friends back home. Despite the grueling schedule, I grew close to the other soldiers in my company. We would commiserate together over the terrible food, share stories about our lives back home, and complain about the lack of... well, about the lack of everything. We would talk about what would happen when we went overseas and alternately boast about not being worried or admit that we were terrified.

We formed a bond. We formed a bond and I realized for the first time in my life I belonged. It was strange to belong when I was certain I never would. I guess I belonged because we were all united with one overwhelming and impossible to escape destiny ahead of us.

I served my tour and then served another. It was only after the second tour I felt strong enough to return to a world that didn't seem as accepting of me as the world of the army. I get home and went to college and lived my life. It's strange because when my army buddies and I get together these days, which ones are still around, anyway, I'm always struck by how the primary lesson I learned through all of it was that I didn't have to please everyone around me. I didn't have to be anyone other than myself to fit in. I just had to be me and the friendships and acquaintances would either come or they wouldn't.

They came, of course, and over the years I've had friendship and love far deeper than that scrawny kid could ever have dreamed possible back in 1968.

Graham Crackers

I imagine most people would be surprised to know that graham crackers are the reason I turned out to be a neurosurgeon. It may sound like a strange correlation but let me explain.

Growing up in the 1980s, my family was not wealthy. We lived in a small apartment in the city and our meals were typically simple and cost-effective. However, one night a week, my mother would make a special treat for dessert. Most people ate the treat (and still do) while camping. S'mores made from graham crackers, marshmallows, and chocolate was a rare sweet indulgence and always a bit of welcome weekly excitement.

As a child, I was fascinated by the intricacies of medical science. The thought of being able to help people heal and feel better seemed like such an incredible gift. Despite my love for biology and anatomy, I was never considered a success at school. Everybody, me included, imagined I'd end up working at a factory or another blue collar job. There was nothing shameful or wrong about those jobs, I didn't think, but the idea of being more seemed out of reach, and that stung. I struggled with standardized tests and often felt discouraged by my grades. A lot of that, I knew, was that I felt uncomfortable in school. I had clothes from the thrift store and rarely had anything new.

But then everything changed early in my freshman year when a friend experienced a traumatic brain injury due to a car accident. I was there when a drunk driver rammed into his car as he was getting out of it right in front of my apartment building. Somehow, I finagled my way into riding in the ambulance with him and I was there at the emergency room. Seeing how doctors and nurses worked together to save his life was a transformative experience. From that moment on, I knew that being a surgeon was my calling.

I swept up the corner store in exchange for a two dollar notebook that I turned into a homework planner. I told myself I couldn't have my weekly s'mores treat unless all my homework was done. I may not have had the discipline to live up to my goal but when I started, I told my mother about my plans. You better believe if my homework wasn't done, I didn't get the marshmallowy, chocolate graham goodness!

I graduated with a 3.5 grade point average. It wasn't the straight A result I wanted but it changed my outlook. I went to community college and got an associate degree there in biology. That time, I earned perfect marks. I still lived at home. I still received no s'more if my work wasn't done. I went to state university after that and this time, I had a scholarship because of my grades in junior college. For the next two years, I worked hard. I still lived at home and I still had to get all of my work done in order to get my treat.

I managed to get accepted into a top medical school. However, my insecurities still lingered. Medical school was four states away from home. I couldn't shake the feeling that I wasn't smart enough or prepared enough to tackle such an intimidating profession. I had a tuition scholarship and my aunt and uncle lived only forty-five minutes away from the school so I had a place to stay. I moved in over the summer. I got a part-time job at a grocery store to help pay my way and not be a burden to my relatives.

The first week of school felt like a nightmare. The insecurities grew stronger and I just didn't think I could make it. On Friday night, while stocking the shelves at the store, I ended up stocking graham crackers. I came home with two boxes, a couple of big chocolate bars, and a package of marshmallows.

The next day, I made s'mores for everyone. My aunt and uncle were delighted, and suddenly, I felt a sense of comfort and assurance flood over me. It reminded me of all the times I enjoyed this before moving to go to medical school. It reminded me that I was the same Jason who got good grades in high school and perfect marks in junior college.

I was the same Jason who earned a scholarship to the state university and a partial scholarship to medical school. I wasn't different now but just in a different location.

In that very moment, I realized that it's the little things in life that can make a big difference. Just like how a simple treat could bring so much happiness to my family in tough times, sometimes the smallest moments of joy can propel us forward to achieve great things. I told my aunt and uncle I'd be making the graham cracker goodness every week for us and they, of course, had no problem with that.

I didn't make a rule for myself about no s'mores until my work was done. I didn't need to. With renewed confidence, I spent long hours in the lab and hospitals, soaking up every bit of knowledge I could. I worked hard at school and I worked hard at my part time job, listening to audio versions of my textbooks while I stocked or cleaned the aisles.

It all paid off and I became a neurosurgeon. I have had the honor of helping countless patients regain their health and live fulfilling lives. I've had the privilege of being like those professionals who helped Marcus all those years ago.

And it's all because of graham crackers.

Now, whenever I feel overwhelmed or stressed, I reach for a graham cracker. It's a small reminder that even in the face of adversity, there is always something to be grateful for. And it's a reminder that anything is possible, as long as you believe in yourself and work hard toward your goals. I still make s'mores every month or so, and I imagine I'll make them for the rest of my life.

High School Chemistry

The day I played Juliet in the school play, I kissed the boy playing Romeo for real. It wasn't something I had planned or even thought of before, but in the heat of the moment, it just felt right. We were both caught up in the romance of the scene, swept away by the passion of our characters.

After we finished the play, I felt a bit embarrassed about what had happened. I wasn't sure how to reconcile my unexpected behavior with Jeremy with my own shyness and uncertainty. As I walked back to my dressing room, I noticed that there was a different atmosphere with the cast. In rehearsal, people seemed a little concerned but now, after the big night, people were smiling and applauding, congratulating us on a job well done.

It was then that I realized that what had happened on stage was something special, something that everyone could feel. It wasn't just about me and my co-star; it was about the magic that Jeremy and I created together, the way that we had transported the audience to a different time and place. And in that moment, I felt proud of what I had accomplished and grateful for the experience that I had been given.

And I liked the kiss.

We did the play for three performances, and I kissed him for real every time. I think the anticipation added to the magic and made it even better. When the play ended, though, I felt more confused than ever.

I'd never thought about the boy in any romantic way before that moment. In fact, for all three performances, when he was Romeo and I was Juliet; I was madly in love with him. When the curtain fell, though, I never gave it much thought.

Over the next few weeks, though, I struggled to make sense of my feelings. I was unsure if I wanted to pursue a relationship with my co-star, or if what had happened between us was just part of the play.

As for Jeremy, he seemed distant and withdrawn. Of course, we barely knew each other before we did the play together and didn't really run in the same circles. He may have just been behaving like he always did and I might have just interpreted it all as him being withdrawn.

The play was a huge hit, though. The first night, we got the typical parents and teachers and students. Someone from the newspaper showed up, though, and he gave us a glowing review so we sold out the last two performances. He wrote, "The chemistry between Alice North and Jeremy King is remarkable and will convince you Romeo and Juliet are real and live right here in town."

Admission money always went to different clubs so the drama program and the French Club both got some funds. Everyone was grateful and it was the first time any event at the high school intended for the general public ever sold out.

It was a fun time and things seemed wonderful except for me growing more and more anxious about my relationship with my Jeremy or, more accurately, my desire for one. I didn't want to come across as needy or obsessive, but I also didn't want to let go of the possibility of something more. It was a delicate balance, and one that I was struggling to find.

Then one day, Jeremy called me out of the blue. He said he had been thinking about maybe getting into acting as a career and wondered if I would get together with him to talk about it.

He was lying.

It turned out that he had been feeling just as confused as I had been. He had enjoyed kissing me on stage and felt something special, but he was

35

afraid I wouldn't feel the same way. He wanted to meet with me just to find out how much of what happened on stage was acting and how much wasn't.

Well, the truth was it was all acting when it happened. All of my feelings for him came after the play was over. You can bet I wasn't going to tell him that, though. I told him I felt something special during the play and I still felt it. The relief on his face was profound.

At that point, I didn't know anything about him and he didn't know anything about me. We'd done a play together and that was it. Somehow, though, we felt a connection that was deep and real to us. So, we set about getting to know things about each other. He was nothing like me at all. We had absolutely nothing in common other than that play.

But it worked.

For some reason, the relationship worked.

Almost forty years later, we still know our lines and every now and then we say them to each other just for fun.

The day I played Juliet in the school play, I kissed the boy playing Romeo for real.

And I still do.

The Coyote

Even though I knew the thing was dangerous for our sheep, and even though I knew my father would be angry with me; I just couldn't bring myself to shoot the coyote when I saw it through my rifle scope. It wasn't like I had anything against hunting. I had been raised on this farm and I'd taken my share of deer, wild pigs, and just about every game bird available. I wasn't against hunting at all. Nonetheless, something about the coyote was different, almost magical.

It wasn't that the coyote wasn't suitable food. There was plenty of justification for killing an animal in order to protect other animals or to protect people or, in this case, their livelihood. It was something different. As I stared at the creature, I couldn't bring myself to shoot it. Instead, I aimed low and squeezed the trigger, sending up a shower of dirt directly in front of its face. It leapt back and disappeared into the trees. It wouldn't remain in the trees but would most certainly return.

My father, who had inherited the farm from his father before him, always taught us that coexisting with nature was the key to farming. I remember the many times he sat us down and explained why we needed to respect nature and work with it, not against it. We hunted enough to have our food secured and we worked the land so that it was never depleted, moving our vegetable garden annually between three plots so each plot remained fallow for two years. We rotated twenty-acre pastures for the sheep as well so they never ate down to the dirt.

Respecting nature meant respecting that there were predators as well as prey and respecting that we often played the role of predator. Respecting nature meant respecting our nature as well. There was no moral reason for me to avoid killing that coyote.

But I couldn't.

It may sound strange, but as I looked at the coyote, there was an energy in its eyes that mesmerized me. It was nothing like I had ever seen before. The way it leaped gracefully over rocks, the way it hunted and ran, there was a sense of freedom and power in its movements that captivated me. I knew I couldn't shoot it, not after seeing it that way.

I walked back to the farmhouse, confused but also oddly excited. Something inside of me had shifted, and the world around me seemed different. My mother stood in the kitchen preparing dinner, saw me and smiled. "I need to put the rifle away," I said with a nervous smile.

"Is everything okay, Honey?" she asked.

I had never been one to speak up when I was confused, but this didn't feel right keeping to myself. "Let me put the gun away and come back."

She nodded and I could see the concern in her face. I quickly added, "It's not a bad thing, Mom. It's just confusing."

She smiled, reassured, and I walked quickly to my room. I unloaded the rifle, just as I was taught, and put the shells in the drawer by my nightstand. I put the rifle on the top shelf of my closet, just as I was taught. Before I stowed it safely away, I wiped it down with an oiled cloth, just as I was taught. One shot didn't require a full cleaning but I seriously considered cleaning it anyway just to delay the conversation with Mom. I stood for a minute or two before finally shaking my head and walking back to the kitchen. She was just putting a roast in the oven, and even now it looked appetizing.

I told her about the coyote and how I couldn't shoot it. She listened intently, nodding slowly before asking if she could tell me a story.

"When I was a little girl, I saw a snow-white bird, a snowy owl, in our fields one winter. I had never seen anything so beautiful in my life, and I was so entranced by it that I refused to shoot it."

"But Mom," I interrupted. "Why would anyone shoot an owl? I guess if you were raising rabbits but owls are... I don't understand."

"Owls kill chickens, honey. I saw a bird of prey and thought I was supposed to kill it. I couldn't, though."

"Well," I said, "You were always doing chores around the farm, you never really had time to play around or stare at birds."

"I suppose that's true," she said with a chuckle. "But sometimes you can get so caught up in the little things you forget to look around and take notice of the beauty around you."

What she had said made sense but I still felt conflicted. My instinct was to protect my father's livelihood, the sheep. My mother must have sensed my confusion because she said, "So what if you didn't shoot the coyote? I didn't kill the owl. I didn't do it just because the owl was beautiful. That's it. Of course, it was illegal to kill them. I didn't know that at the time. I found out when I told my father I saw an owl and lied to him. I told him I tried to hit it and missed."

I smiled and said, "You were a bad girl. Next time you catch me lying I'm going to remind you of this."

She smiled and said, "Nope. I was only nine years old. You're almost seventeen. You know better."

"But what are we going to tell Dad?" I asked.

Mom said, "We're going to tell him all about your ideas about how to protect the sheep without having to worry about keeping guard for the coyotes."

"But Mom," I said, "I don't have any ideas!"

"Really?" she asked. Then she shrugged, "Well, you better come up with some. That roast will be done in an hour and forty-five minutes and we'll be eating dinner ten minutes later."

My mother's words sparked a new sense of purpose in me and I rushed to my room and sat down with some paper to brainstorm. These days, I guess someone would just go on the Internet to get answers and ideas. That wasn't possible back then. In any case, I came up with ten different ideas and at dinner I was surprised at how impressed my father was with some of them. Within six months, we had new fencing, some noisemakers that went off at random times, and two more sheepdog guardians.

The changes on the farm didn't seem as powerful as the changes in me. As time went by, I began to see the world through a different lens. I started noticing things that I had never seen before. I noticed how the leaves on the trees turned golden yellow before falling to the ground, and how the sunflowers swayed in the wind. I saw the beauty in everything around me, not just the things that were familiar to me. Not too many years later, I moved away to the city to pursue my studies. However, the lessons I learned on the farm stayed with me. I like to think I approach life like I ended up approaching the situation with the coyote, with a little creativity, hard work, and an open mind.

Several years ago, I returned to the farm for my father's 80th birthday celebration. It was a heartwarming reunion, and I could see that many things had changed, but in many ways, everything was still the same. As I walked around the fields, I saw my great nephew, my brother's grandson, positioned with his rifle.

When he saw me, he put his rifle down and ran to me. "Aunt Amelia!" he cried as he hugged me.

"Would you like me to tell you a story your great grandmother told me?" I asked.

I told him about the Snowy Owl. As I finished telling the story, I looked into his eyes and saw the same fascination and bewilderment that I imagine my mother saw in my eyes all those years before. I told him about the coyote, and I could see that I had made an impact, and that the lesson I had learned through my experience was worth sharing.

Even today, when someone asks me how I became the person I am, I always recount the story of the coyote and how I learned that sometimes, there were solutions beyond the obvious. I guess it's not all that impressive a story as stories go but it was very profound for me. It was a powerful lesson then and it remains one now. To this day, the conversation and the direction to come up with alternative solutions is the memory of my mother that feels the most vivid and powerful. I often think of how that one decision to shoot in front of the coyote because I couldn't bring myself to kill it changed my perspective on everything that happed afterward.

A Real Tragedy

When I walked into my sister's bedroom, I found her and my best friend together without a stitch of clothing on, and my first inclination was to throw Tom out of the window. They both looked at me, red-faced and ashamed, and I knew right away that I couldn't do that. There had to be a better way to handle the situation.

I stormed out of the room, feeling betrayed and confused. My sister and I were very close, and Tom had been my closest friend since childhood. I couldn't believe they would do something like this behind my back. For days, I avoided them both, seething with anger and hurt.

It took a while but as time went on, I began to realize that my anger wasn't helping anyone - least of all me. I needed to find a way to move past this and forgive them both. My sister and I avoided each other although we'd shared a home since my parents retired. Things were tense but one day, I finally called Tom and asked him to come over. I told my sister I wanted to talk. When all three of us were in the same place, they both looked nervous.

We sat down together in the living room, and I began to speak. At first, my words were harsh and accusatory, but as I spoke, I began to soften. I told them how much their actions had hurt me, but I also said that I didn't want to lose either of them.

My sister began to cry, apologizing profusely for what they had done. She told me how sorry she was and how she regretted it deeply. In that moment, something shifted. I felt my anger dissipate, replaced by an overwhelming sense of love and understanding. I realized that holding onto this grudge was not only hurting them, but it was also hurting me.

My friend, on the other hand, looked at me like I was an idiot. Tom said, "How much?"

"What do you mean?" I asked.

"I didn't understand that you owned Sandy. I didn't know she was your property. So how much for me to buy her from you so I can give her back her freedom and she can make her own decisions about her life."

I stared at him in shock and I couldn't pretend I wasn't angry as can be. I think it was made worse for me because my sister stared at Tom like he was some kind of magical hero after he said those words. I know I was also angry because there was truth in what he said. I'd definitely behaved as though Sandra had no agency of her own. I think sometimes anger burns hotter when there's truth in an accusation. I was so angry, I think things might have come to blows but instead, we were hit by another blow.

A knock on my door revealed my neighbor, Robert. He needed me to feed his dogs for a week because he had to go to the city hospital. Why? Well, that was the other blow.

In fact, it was a devastating blow for the whole community. A young girl, only ten years old, had been diagnosed with leukemia. Her name was Emily, and she was our neighbor's daughter. Emily's diagnosis shook our town to its core. Everyone knew her. I guess in a town like ours, everyone pretty much knew everyone. Emily, though, was the kind of girl who lit up a room with her infectious smile and sparkling eyes.

I felt helpless in the face of it all. I also felt stupid. I'd been so devastated and hurt because two people I loved decided to take their relationship to a deeper place. How foolish that seemed now that a true tragedy struck the town. How powerfully resounded Tom's words about my attitude toward my sister's right to make her own choices! It seemed foolish and stupid to be angry and hurt when something far more real and far more devastating suddenly fell into our lap.

The first day, I not only fed the dogs but Tom, Sandra and I did housecleaning, did all the yardwork, and went to the grocery store so Robert, his wife, and Emily would come home to full cabinets. We also

43

bought some toys and books for Emily and filled the house with flowers. We used money we'd saved for our annual vacation together.

That's when my sister came up with an idea. She suggested that we organize a fundraiser to help Emily and her family pay for medical expenses. Tom and I didn't know how much of a difference we could make but my sister was determined, and we agreed to help.

We put our heads together and came up with a plan. We would organize a charity walk-a-thon, where people would pledge money for every mile walked. We would start at the park and walk through our town, spreading awareness about leukemia and raising funds for Emily at the same time. Just to ensure the walk-a-thon route covered fifteen miles, we would have to cross through town three times. It was a daunting task, but we knew we had to try. We spent the week they were gone planning it all and got local businesses involved.

When Robert and Emily returned, we shared our plans and with their agreement began promoting it. Emily went through times when she was her normal bright self and times when she was very weak and small. Every day when I went to work, I bought something for her like a comic book or a little doll. Stopping by her house before going to mine became the standard.

On the day of the walk, the turnout was incredible. Almost a thousand people showed up, most of them from out of town. I guess there was some news coverage in the city. We all wore t-shirts emblazoned with Emily's name. We set off on our route, passing by homes and storefronts decorated with signs of support and encouragement.

It was on the walk that Tom told me he was marrying Sandra. I guess he thought I would be angry and hurt again. I congratulated him and hugged my sister. We raised almost fifty thousand dollars for Emily and we got enough news coverage that there were some big corporations and philanthropists that agreed to cover the rest.

Tom and Sandra got married and I was Tom's best man. Emily was a flower girl even though she wasn't able to walk by that time. I'd like to tell you I never tried to make decisions for my sister again but if I told you that, it would be a lie. I certainly got better about accepting her right to decide things for herself.

Emily got better, too. She went through chemo, radiation, and a bone marrow transplant. It was a long road, filled with ups and downs, but she fought with all her might. I spent almost three years bringing her books, candy bars, little toys, and flowers every day after work. In the end, she won. She beat leukemia, finished school, went to college, became a pediatrician, and had children of her own. Every few months, I get a letter or a card in the mail from her and when she's feeling funny, she'll send me a comic book or a candy bar.

As for Tom and Sandra, they still live in my little hometown, just a few blocks from me. Tom's still my best friend and my sister still makes her own decisions. I often think about how that might all have been lost if not for a real tragedy replacing one of my own making. It's funny how life works out, isn't it?

Overgrown Branches

My neighbor and I finally made peace about the tree trimming on the day the Challenger exploded after takeoff. It was a moment that changed everything for me, and it made me see things in a completely different way. It was 1986, and I was living in Florida at the time. I had been having problems with my neighbor over a tree that was blocking our view. We had been arguing about it for weeks, and we just couldn't seem to come to an agreement. But all of that changed on that fateful day.

I remember watching the Challenger take off from Cape Canaveral. It was a beautiful day, and the sun was shining brightly. The whole world seemed to be watching as the shuttle blasted off into space. I watched from my backyard and we were excited enough that our typical bickering about the branches that would fill my yard with leaves and who was responsible for trimming them was set aside for the launch. We were all so excited but then everything went horribly wrong.

My neighbor and I were standing in our backyards, staring up at the sky when we heard a loud explosion. At first, we thought it was thunder, and it was surreal. We saw the explosion in the sky but it was so far away, we couldn't accept what we saw. We knew something terrible had happened, and we knew what it was but we didn't want to know and so our heads came up with a million other reasons.

My neighbor didn't have a television set and I didn't bat an eye when he stepped through the gate between our backyards. We rushed inside to turn on the news, hoping there would be none, hoping we were entirely wrong.

We weren't.

Details came in over the next several hours but there was really only one detail that mattered. The Challenger had exploded, killing all seven crew members aboard. My neighbor remained at my house to stay close to the television set. It never occurred to me to think twice about it. We ordered food and kept our eyes glued to the television screen.

That moment changed everything for me. Suddenly, the argument with my neighbor over the tree seemed foolish and meaningless. Who cared about the view on any particular day? It didn't just change things for me and my neighbor. It changed things far more universally for me. I remember growing up a teacher told me almost everyone her age could tell you exactly where she was and what she was doing when John F. Kennedy was assassinated.

I knew this was my generation's event, the one where everyone I met who was my age would know exactly where she was and what she was doing when the Challenger exploded. When we finally turned off the television, my neighbor said, "I'll get that stupid tree trimmed tomorrow. I wanted it trimmed but just didn't want to lose the fight."

I laughed and said, "I don't even care if it gets trimmed anymore. If you do, though, I'll pay for half."

I guess we both realized that we had been acting like children, bickering over something that wasn't really important. It seemed particularly unimportant when I learned the cost to have it trimmed turned out to be less than twenty-five dollars. My half was less than we spent on the food while we watched the news. We weren't fighting because of any effort that we'd want to put out. Just like my neighbor, I wanted to win.

If this were a Hollywood movie, I guess this is the part where I'd tell you my neighbor and I became good friends and eventually started a wonderful romance, got married, and have been married for thirty-years or so. Well, it didn't happen at all. We never really became friends but we stopped being enemies. I could count on him if I went on vacation to water my yard or take care of my houseplants. He could count on me for the same.

We were at peace.

We were at peace because a terrible event taught us that silly arguments based on ego have no place in a happy life. I like to think the terrible event taught me a number of lessons about living in peace that I carry with me to this day.

Come Back to Me

It wasn't hard for seventeen-year-old me to get a college boy to buy beer back in 1968. There was talk about lowering the drinking age to eighteen but that was a year off for me and we were all pretty sure it wouldn't happen until we were well past twenty-one anyway. As for the college kids, it was almost like a rite of passage when you turned twenty-one that you'd be picking up beer for friends or for any pretty girl who asks. There I was, a pretty high school girl, doing all I could to join in on the fun.

It was always a little awkward when the boy found out the six packs were for me to enjoy with my boyfriend and our friends and this particular pretty girl wasn't interested in a date with an older guy. They might have groaned about it but there were no hard feelings. Hey, it was the sixties and we were rebelling against the norm, high school kids included.

My boyfriend, Mark, was a cool dude. He had long hair and a guitar and he played in a band. We'd been together since junior high school, and we were inseparable. Our group of friends was made up of rebels and oddballs, and we loved each other for who we were. We spent most nights hanging out at someone's house, listening to music, and getting high or buzzed.

And then it happened.

Mark got a letter in the mail that said he had been drafted. We couldn't believe it. We all knew people who had gone off to war but it was different when it was someone close to you. Mark was devastated and so was I. We had never talked about what would happen if he got drafted. It was like we both thought it would never happen. We were rebels and we were oddballs but we weren't political. We were hippies only when it came to smoking grass and living our high school version of free love. We weren't protestors or even conscientious about anything, much less objections.

The next few weeks were a blur. We spent as much time together as possible, trying to make the most of the little time we had left. We talked about everything we could think of and tried to figure out what the future held for us. One night, we sat on the hood of his car looking up at the stars. Mark started playing his guitar and singing a song he wrote for me.

"Come back to me, my love

when you're far away.

I'll be waiting here

for you to come and stay"

I cried the whole time he played. It was like he was saying goodbye without actually saying it. We knew that once he left for basic training, things would never be the same.

And we were right.

The day he left, I felt like I was in a dream. We said goodbye at the airport and I went home alone. My parents tried to console me but I didn't want to talk to them. I didn't want to talk to anyone. Of course, I didn't have much of a choice because all my friends wanted to console me, too, and when they showed up, my mom got right to work getting us snacks and food and telling everyone to call their parents so they could stay the night. My mom set up the guest room for the boys and sleeping bags in my room for the girls. We spent the whole night talking about Mark and how much we were going to miss him. We promised to write to him every week and send him care packages filled with all his favorite snacks. I suppose that cheered me up. Maybe more importantly, it gave me my own plan to follow.

In the weeks that followed, we kept our promise. We all wrote letters filled with details of our lives and sent packages with pictures of ourselves and little trinkets that reminded us of him. It was our way of staying connected and letting him know that he was loved and missed.

But as the months went by, things started to change. The news from Vietnam was getting worse and the death toll was rising. It was hard to keep up hope when the reality of the war was so grim. Our group of friends started to drift apart and we stopped hanging out as much. We were all scared and uncertain of what the future held.

They stopped coming over to make care packages. They stopped writing letters.

I didn't. I wrote to him every day and I started working weekends at my father's paint store so I could keep sending him care packages. My parents were so impressed with my change in behavior and me losing my wild streak that they always helped out with boxes, items for the care package, and postage. I graduated high school and stopped working at the paint store because one of the clients, a builder, offered me a full time job at his office.

So, I worked full time, went to the community college in the evenings, and kept things going with Mark. I wrote to him every day and sent care packages every weekend. Mark wrote me back sporadically but it never seemed like enough and it was worse because I always got the letters weeks after he wrote them. After almost a year of that, I began to give up hope. I still wrote to him. I still sent the care packages. I did it numbly, out of habit. I guess I convinced myself Mark would be a casualty and I would never see him again. Maybe I kept writing just so I wouldn't be devastated by guilt when I got the notice he was gone.

But one day, everything changed again. I got a letter from Mark saying that he was coming home. His tour had ended and he would be back in a few weeks. I couldn't believe it. It was like a weight had been lifted off my shoulders. I didn't even finish the letter but rushed to my parents to ask them to help me throw a big party to welcome him home. That's when my dad looked at the letter and told me it was sixteen days old. He was arriving in the morning! There was even flight information.

My parents and I waited with signs and balloons, ready to welcome him home. There were a few friends who came, too, and even though I felt like they didn't deserve to be there after they stopped writing and sending packages, I was too happy to say anything. When he finally walked through the gate, it was like something out of a movie. I ran to him and hugged him so tightly! It was like nothing else mattered in that moment.

Well, we got married the next day.

We didn't have to elope. Mom and Dad shut down the paint store and drove us to the courthouse. Since they weren't paying for a wedding, they worked with Mark's parents and got us a down payment on a house. We were inseparable again and we'd somehow gone from teen rebels to young citizens. Looking back on that time now, I realize how much we learned about love and resilience. We faced some of the toughest challenges but we never gave up. We kept pushing forward and supporting each other every step of the way. It wasn't always easy, but we never lost hope.

That era of the 60s was a time of great change and upheaval but for me and Mark, it was also a time of community and togetherness. I kept working at the builder's and finished at the community college. Mark worked at a metal fabrication company and went to night school. We built a life together, a good life.

He still played his guitar and every weekend for years I watched his perform at a little bar, sipping a beer while the man I loved entertained the people there. I often thought about how obtaining a beer wasn't an adventure anymore and not all that important to me. All of my high school friends are just acquaintances now, people I used to know, used to party with, and used to get high with while we listened to music.

Mark and I, though, are still together and every now and then, just for kicks, I'll make a care package for him just like the ones I used to send him when he was overseas, sweet love letters and all.

Town Pariah

I didn't always behave growing up but I didn't burn down Martin Nelson's shack like everyone thought I did. It was the mid-1960s, and life was tough for everyone in our small town. No one knew why Martin's shack burned to the ground, but everyone pointed their fingers at me just because I'd walked through his yard a week before and he'd yelled at me and let his dog loose. I had to run across the street and jump a fence just to get away.

I didn't do it by the blamed me. It was hard not to feel downtrodden because of the incident. The townsfolk shunned me. I went from just being a kid in town to being a troublemaker in their eyes. They decided I'd end up in jail or prison one day. They decided I was a blight on the town and it hurt. My father told me not to let their unkind words and cold stares get to me. He told me not to allow them to dictate who I was or who I was going to be. He especially said it would be easy to let them turn me into the person they already thought I was.

One day, my fortunes changed when I signed up for the school's debate team. It felt like it was now or never, do or die. It was an opportunity for me to break free from my trashy image, to show the world that there was more to me than meets the eye. On the other hand, I knew it was probably a fool's errand. Mrs. Edna, our English teacher, was responsible for choosing the students to represent our school for the statewide tournament. I was sure that neither she nor anyone else would pick me, given my reputation in town. But Mrs. Edna had other ideas.

She saw how hard I worked, how diligent I was about researching the topics we were debating, and how well I presented my arguments. In other words, she saw something in me that most people in town did not, she saw potential. I was one of the students chosen for the team, and, as a result, I got judges talking about me for all the right reasons. Soon, it became apparent that my decision to join the debating team was one of the best things that ever happened to me.

We won every round of the tournament, thanks to my quick wits and ability to articulate even the most complex concepts with clarity. And just like that, I had become someone different in the eyes of many. There was a newfound respect for me and the work that I had put in; although it was still difficult being around some of the folks in town. Even the ones who respected me thought I'd turned myself around. I was still guilty of burning down that shack, to them, but I'd managed to somehow get my life on track.

We were a tiny town, though, and any success on a large scale, even with a debate team, was a point of dramatic pride. I kept winning, too. I won the tournaments leading up to the state finals and won the state finals, too. Due to that fearlessness that had helped me to take on the debate team notwithstanding the sense of impending doom and lack of faith in myself, I found new strength. I began to come out of my shell, and with each passing day, I gained more confidence in myself. My grades went from average to perfect, and even the holdouts in town admitted I was a good kid... now.

I was trusted.

In the beginning of my freshman year of high school, people wanted nothing to do with me. In my junior year, a number of people in town offered me part time jobs. All the while, almost everyone still believed I burned down the shack. It just didn't seem to matter to anyone anymore. After all, Martin had insurance and his place was rebuilt so nobody would call it a shack anymore but a nice little house. It was a bad thing to do but somehow it had all worked out for the best.

I'd long since given up protesting that I hadn't done the deed. Since nobody cared about it anymore, everyone always seemed very patronizing and condescending about that.

They treated me like I had to somehow hold onto that and they let me proclaim my innocence with long-suffering, tolerant expressions on their faces. It felt maddening but, of course, there wasn't a thing I could do about it.

And the truth of the matter was pretty simple. Everyone was probably right not to care. I'd gone from being a nobody to the town pariah to the favorite son. When I graduated from high school, I got scholarship awards from the Rotary Club and two different lodges. Because of my success on the debate team, those scholarships weren't even necessary. A college recruited me and paid for all four years, room and board included. So, I got to use the little scholarships just for spending money.

On the day I was accepted into law school, my mother gave me a call. She had an interesting story to tell me. Martin Nelson had "got religion." He gave up drinking and smoking and took down all his *no trespassing* signs. He also took out a mortgage on his house because he wanted to pay his insurance company back. He confessed in church that he'd burned his shack down himself one night while drunk. For almost eight years, people believed I'd been a young punk and taken revenge with violence. Suddenly, I was vindicated.

I returned home a few weeks later to spend the summer with my parents before I left for law school. You know what happened?

Nothing.

Nobody treated me differently because the absolute truth was that nobody cared if I'd done it. Sure, we were a tiny town and there was gossip and there were a lot of apologies to me but there was nobody left who still treated me poorly so nobody had to change behavior. I think back on the situation often and realize my life became something fulfilling, effective, and happy because of a false accusation. Somehow, being the towns pariah turned me into a successful lawyer.

I find it helpful now because I get to tell this story to my clients when they're dealing with accusations made about them. The truth is, what people say about us or blame us for, how they characterize our lives, is a lot less important than what we decide to do with the life given to us.

The Edge of Seventeen

Twelve days before my seventeenth birthday, I went camping in the middle of the desert all by myself. It was something I had been planning to do for months. As a teenager living in the 1970s, newly exposed to something people called cosmic consciousness and world awareness, I felt the need to break free from the confines of my small town and discover what the world had in store for me.

As I set up my tent, I looked around at the vast expanse of sand and rocks. There was not a single soul in sight, and the silence was deafening. I felt a sense of liberation that I had never experienced before. I built a campfire and made myself some soup, listening to music on my transistor radio. As the night fell, I gazed at the stars, and the sky seemed to stretch out forever. I felt as though I could reach out and touch them, and for the first time in my life, I felt like nothing was impossible.

The next day, I decided to go on a hike to explore the barren wilderness. I packed some snacks and water and headed out into the unknown. The sun was beating down on me, and the wind was picking up, but I kept going. The more I walked, the more I felt a sense of independence and self-discovery. As I climbed a rocky outcropping, I looked back at the desert below me. The view was breathtaking, and it made me realize how small my problems and fears were in the grand scheme of things.

Of course, it seemed like everything was small in the grand scheme of things.

And every thought, no matter how mundane, seemed filled with importance. I looked over the desert and even realizing I didn't care too much for yogurt seemed like some kind of intense revelation.

That night, I sat by the fire again, reflecting on my journey. I thought about how I had always felt like an outsider and how I longed to find my place in the world.

I came to the conclusion that being alone in the desert made me realize that I didn't need to fit in with anyone else's expectations. The only one I needed to please was me. It was the first of about a dozen life-transforming decisions I made during that trip.

At the edge of seventeen, everything seemed significant, especially when I was in the middle of the desert and there were no distractions at all that forced a little grounding on me. My last day in the desert, created a rockpile about two feet high. I built it around a mayonnaise jar. In the jar, I placed my watch as a statement that my time was my own and my compass because I was going to choose my own direction!

After a week, I returned to my hometown feeling rejuvenated and motivated. I started to explore different activities and hobbies that I had never tried before. I joined a theatre group and discovered a newfound passion for acting. It lasted a month or so before I discovered a newfound passion for rock collecting.

See, of all my life-transforming decisions made there in the desert, I only remembered one. I was going to be my own man.

So, I hopped from passion to passion because I had no idea who this man I was going to become actually was.

Theatre.

Rock collecting.

Macrame.

Sand candles.

Poetry.

Flower arranging.

I jumped from passion to passion and somehow convinced myself it was all about being certain that the only person whose expectations mattered was me.

As time passed, I graduated from high school and moved to the city for college. I couldn't pick a major yet because I was passionate about archeology for a week and then passionate about communications. I ended up undeclared and when I got a degree, it was in liberal arts, which is another way to say I couldn't decide on anything.

But I was my own man!

And I had never felt so unfulfilled in my life.

A few weeks after graduating, I bought a pup tent and a camp stove and headed back to the desert. I guess I thought when I got there, I would somehow reconnect with all the wonder and joy of being young and experiencing dramatic intellectual and spiritual upheaval.

Instead, I looked at the sand and the cactus and tried to understand why I'd thought a place so barren was so beautiful. I didn't even leave the campsite the first day but just sat there feeling directionless and unhappy.

I was my own man and I was unhappy with the man I was.

The next day, I forced myself to venture out from the camp and found that rock outcropping. I stood at the top waiting for profound revelations that would somehow transform me and illuminate my path. None came. The only thing of any significance was pain at my ankle because I brushed up against a jumping cholla, and that cactus's spines are no fun at all.

I decided to go home the next morning. Directionless and unhappy at home seemed better than directionless and unhappy in the desert. This place had been so important to me back when I was on the edge of seventeen and now, it seemed like everything about my trip was just foolishness.

The next morning, I packed everything up. I felt bitter, confused, and angry.

I got in my car but then, almost as a point of rebellion against the desert and against my immature, melodramatic almost-seventeen feelings, I decided to go find the rock pile and get my watch and my compass from the mayonnaise jar, to undo the last evidence of my stupidity. So, I made one more trek.

I almost didn't recognize the rock pile. It was larger. The mayonnaise jar was gone, replaced by a trunk-sized metal lockbox painted black. It had a combination lock but painted in block letters on the top of that lockbox was a surprising message.

IF YOU NEED HELP, THE COMBINATION IS 14L 23R 8L

Well, I didn't need help but I certainly had to find out what was in that lockbox! I opened the lock and opened the box and inside saw the mayonnaise jar, my watch, and my compass. I saw a lot more, too. There was a first aid kit. There was a wool blanket. There was a map to an oasis four miles away. There were flares and matches and there were several pamphlets about survival in the desert.

There was a laminated piece of paper explaining the box. It turns out a couple went hiking in the desert and got lost. They couldn't find their way home until they happened upon this rockpile and found the compass left for them by somehow who cared enough to think of people in trouble. They used the compass to get to safety and then returned a month later with the lockbox. It said if you needed anything, you were welcome to it but someday return with a replacement and something new.

Their new item was the lockbox and the blanket.

Everything else in that box came from others who had been helped by it. Inside was a journal for people to record their interactions with the location and I counted six people who had been helped by it along with one person who hadn't needed anything but had returned with the survival pamphlets.

I guess the answers I sought were here. Everywhere we go, we leave a mark. I kept searching for direction but never once thought about what I left behind. There will come a time (closer now than when I was just shy of seventeen) when all that remains of me is what I leave behind. I'd been so busy trying to decide how to live my life that I'd forgotten I was already living it.

I walked back to my car and got my tent and my camp stove. I put them in the lockbox and wrote a note in the journal.

I came to the desert for answers to my questions and you gave me the help I needed.

I'd expected a glorious, transformative revelation that would resound to the Heavens the way the sight of the desert resounded in my mind all those years ago. Instead, as I drove away, I felt a quiet serenity, a certainty that things were exactly as they should be.

The Amazon Princess and the Runaways

I guess I felt a little bit jealous when Henry Summers asked Helen, my next-door neighbor, to the fall dance. It stung but the jealousy didn't last because that night a new television show premiered and from then on, I could only give my heart to Diana Prince and the woman who played her, Lynda Carter.

I don't mean give my heart to Wonder Woman the way I wanted to give my heart to Henry. I mean I gave it to her in an entirely different way.

Growing up in suburban America during the 1970s was both magical and challenging, especially for me. As a teenage girl, I struggled with self-doubt and insecurities, compounded by peer pressure and societal expectations. My parents wanted me to study hard, attend college, get a good job, and eventually settle down with a nice boy, preferably from our community. They meant well, but their narrow worldview clashed with my own aspirations and dreams.

Of course, my parents weren't the only ones who had expectations of me. I was really good at math but I didn't enjoy it. Nonetheless, teachers at the school wanted me to take advanced classes and get into engineering or even physics. I didn't like any of that. I didn't want any of that. Some of my friends wanted me to go with them right out of high school. They wanted to move as a group to some town in the Midwest where they wanted to join a commune. It was just another plan that would tell me where I was supposed to be and when I was supposed to be there. Other friends vied for my attention. They wanted me to attend the same college as they did.

The truth was, somewhere around age fifteen, it seemed like everyone wanted my time, attention, and my commitment to a future I didn't necessarily want. I wanted more than just a conventional life.

I wanted to explore the world, see new places, learn all about different cultures, and maybe even write about my adventures someday. How could I make that happen when I felt trapped in this idyllic but suffocating environment?

That's where Wonder Woman came in. From the moment I saw her spin around and transform into her alter-ego, Diana Prince, I was hooked on her bravery, kindness, and intelligence. She was a superhero, yes, but she was also a normal woman who faced everyday challenges with grace and fortitude.

Watching her battle villains, rescue innocents, and stand up for justice inspired me to do the same in my own small way. I started reading books about making a difference and I joined a group of like-minded teenagers who wanted to make a difference in our community. We didn't want to change the world with big protests or giant changes. We thought doing things a little step at a time was the way to do things.

Together, we organized a charity fundraiser for the local animal shelter, volunteered at the food bank, and hosted a fair to get people involved in community gardening and things like that. We faced opposition and criticism from some adults who thought we were too young or idealistic, but we persevered and proved them wrong.

All the while, my life had a soundtrack. In the seventies, there was music for every occasion. From disco to punk, from Motown to rock, there was a sound for every mood and moment. I loved dancing with my friends at school dances, listening to records in my bedroom, and attending concerts whenever I could afford them.

One band that stood out for me was The Runaways. They were an all-female group that rocked hard and defied expectations. They sang about sex, drugs, and rebellion, and they looked cool doing it.

I admired them for their guts and talent, and I saw them as a symbol of empowerment and liberation.

I felt a kinship with lead singer Cherie Currie, who was around my age and struggled to assert herself in a male-dominated industry. I wanted to be like her, fearless and confident, and to find my own voice and style. I even started taking guitar lessons and writing songs, just for myself at first, but eventually for a local band that needed a rhythm guitarist. I wasn't really any good, at least not good enough to be professional but, then again, I also didn't have a magic lasso or bracelets that could stop bullets but I sometimes felt like Wonder Woman. Playing music gave me a sense of purpose and creativity that I had never felt before. It was a way to express my emotions and ideas, and to connect with others. It was also a way to challenge myself and overcome my self-doubt, by learning new chords, practicing for hours, and performing in front of an audience. Looking back, I realized that the 1970s were a turning point in my life, a time when I discovered my own identity and values. Wonder Woman and The Runaways were just two icons that influenced me, but they represented everything about my awakening.

It was a time when young people were asserting themselves. It was a time when people once ignored were demanding equal rights and opportunities. It was a time of experimentation, innovation, and rebellion, when anything seemed possible and everything was worth trying. I explored possibilities and I tried just about everything.

I may not have achieved all of my dreams or lived up to all of my expectations, but I'm proud of what I accomplished and learned during that pivotal decade. I learned to be brave, kind, and smart, like Wonder Woman, and to be bold, creative, and authentic, like The Runaways.

I learned to follow my own path and to challenge the status quo, to stand up for what I believed in and to make a difference in the world. And even though it's been decades since then, I still feel inspired and uplifted by the memories and lessons of the 1970s, and by the timeless message of Wonder Woman: that you can be a hero, too, if you believe in yourself and in the power of love and justice.

The 1974 Mustang

It seemed like the moment I got my first car in the Summer of 1978, I suddenly found myself driving all of my friends everywhere. It was a pea green 1974 Mustang that I bought from a neighbor for five hundred dollars from money saved working at the gas station after school and on weekends, and even though it wasn't the most stylish car on the road, it was mine, and I was proud of it.

At first, I was hesitant to let my friends ride in my car. I didn't want to be responsible for anyone getting hurt, and I didn't want anyone messing up my new ride. But as the summer went on, I realized that my car was more than just a way to get around; it was a ticket to adventure.

One weekend, my best friend Trudy and I decided to take a road trip up to the mountains. We packed a cooler full of sandwiches and soda and set off early in the morning. The drive was beautiful, with winding roads and sweeping vistas. When we got to our destination, we hiked up to a hidden waterfall and swam in the icy pool at its base. It was magical. More than that, it was something we'd just decided we wanted to do and we could do it!

I'd never experienced that kind of thing before. We just talked about how nice it would be and then we did it! This pea green Mustang had become a ticket to experiences and I wanted to enjoy every single last one that I could!

After that trip, I was hooked. My car became a symbol of freedom and possibility. I started taking longer and longer trips, exploring new cities and meeting new people. I even drove across the country one summer, stopping at roadside diners and camping under the stars. I made friends along the way. Sometimes one or two of them would ride along for a few days. Sometimes I stayed at a new friend's house for a few days before that car seemed to call to me to tell me it was time to move on.

That was the summer right after my high school graduation. When I got home, I felt like the world was just alight with possibilities and adventure. I spent six months at home before my next grand adventure would start, my first semester at college. By then, my car and I had already had adventure after adventure together.

But my car wasn't just a source of personal adventure. It also became a way to help others. One day, I was driving through my neighborhood when I saw an elderly man struggling to carry a heavy package. I pulled over and offered him a ride. He was so grateful that he told all of his friends about me. Before long, I was the go-to person in my neighborhood for rides to the grocery store or doctor's appointments.

I mean, it just happened that way.

I guess back in the 1970s, things like that could happen. I'm not so sure those sorts of things could happen today. There might be places left like that. I hope so. I enjoyed all of those errands and all of the smiles so much that I found ways to do the same thing in college. I joined a group of volunteers who drove food and supplies to communities in need. We loaded up our cars and drove minutes into impoverished neighborhoods or sometimes hours to bring relief to people affected by natural disasters.

Looking back on those years, I'm grateful for my little pea green Mustang, but even more grateful for the experiences it brought me. It wasn't just a car; it was a symbol of hope and possibility. It showed me that one person, with small acts of kindness could make a difference in the world. I knew that because the one world that was changed completely by all of this was mine.

I became a different person.

I really liked the person I became.

As I drive a different car now, I remember the adventures I had and the people I met driving around in my first one. I know that those memories will stay with me for the rest of my life.

Even today, as I reflect on those years, I'm inspired by the stories of ordinary people doing extraordinary things. People who saw a need and decided to act, people who took a chance and discovered new opportunities, people who found the courage to follow their dreams.

Whenever I see a young person getting behind the wheel, I always pretend it must be their first car. I smile, knowing the adventures and opportunities that will appear in front of them. I think about how their life will change. I think about all my adventures, too. For me, that little green Mustang was more than just a car. It was a reminder that anything is possible if you're willing to take risks and work hard. It was a lesson that when you're rewarded for that work it's sometimes best to share that reward with others. When I did that, my entire world changed.

On the Shores of Lake Eerie

I spent the summer of 1968 in a cabin on the shores of Lake Eerie obsessed with an older woman, Evelyn Brill, who was already a junior in high school. I was just fourteen and the idea of falling in love seemed glamorous and accessible. As much as I wanted to impress her, I had no clue how to make it happen. It's fair to say, though, that I thought of very little else during that summer.

I spent most of my days observing from the shadows, peeking through the bushes that separated her family's cabin from mine. Evelyn appeared so confident and self-assured; I was in awe of her. I knew I wasn't her type, even though I wanted to be. I was too young for her; too inexperienced, too shy, too immature. But still, I couldn't resist her. Everything about her fascinated me. A day doing nothing but staring at her from a distance was better than a day of doing anything else.

I thought she would never notice me, of course. Girls like her didn't notice boys who were just out of junior high school and not even freshmen yet. One afternoon, though, Evelyn caught me staring. I couldn't look away even though my cheeks felt as hot as could be and I imagined I was bright red with blushing. Instead of laughing or making fun of me, she simply said, "Hi there. I've been meaning to ask you something. There's an ice cream shop at the marina. Do you want to go and get some with me?"

Go with her?

To the marina?

Go with her to the marina to have ice cream?

I was dreaming. That was it. I had to be dreaming. There was no other explanation.

I was hesitant but not because I didn't want to go. I was hesitant because it seemed like right then my voice decided to disappear. I just stared at her, finally understanding what that saying about a deer in the headlights meant. Somehow, I managed to nod and I must have looked like a complete idiot but, again, she just smiled. "Well, let's go, then."

She was just taking the kid next door out for ice cream, I think. As for me, I was going on a date with a beautiful woman! I hurried down to the shore, around the hedge and up into her yard. I bet I ran up to her looking like a kid on Christmas morning running downstairs to open presents. I must have seemed very young and very immature but she didn't make me feel that way at all. On the contrary, she smiled when I got there, took my hand, and said, "I know the way."

She didn't hold my hand like I was a little kid she needed to keep under control. I mean, she didn't hold my hand like I was her boyfriend or anything. She just held it as we walked and she talked animatedly about how much she loved her summers at the lake and how much she loved ice cream and how much fun there was to be had there.

We went to the ice cream shop and she ordered a banana split for both of us and we sat at a table enjoying it. She talked about how what we ate were real, authentic banana splits because it had crushed pineapple and fresh strawberries instead of strawberry sauce. It was the most magical moment of my life.

Up to then.

It seemed like every day following had the most magical moment of my life in it.

The next weeks were magical. We rode bicycles, shared ice cream almost every day, and discussed everything under the sun from classic movies to famous musicians to the civil rights movement unfolding on television.

We fished from the shore while we listened to music and every time I caught a fish, I felt like I was some kind of super man impressing her.

There was absolutely nothing that happened during that summer that didn't feel especially significant. It seemed like every moment had everything to do with Evelyn. She liked fried chicken so fried chicken became my favorite food. She liked Joan Baez, so Joan Baez became my favorite musical act. Her favorite color was green so you can imagine my favorite color.

The summer passed quickly until suddenly I realized I only had a couple more days with her.

A couple more days!

I was fourteen years old in love with an older woman, much older! She was almost seventeen! I was in love with this older woman but she would go home to Maryland and I would go back to Pittsburg. It felt like my life would end, that my only chance for happiness would disappear at the end of August.

I didn't know what to do!

The days didn't pass any more slowly just because I wanted them to. In fact, it seemed like because I wanted it to last, the rest of the time flew by. On our second to last day, Evelyn said, "We have to do something special today, something we'll never forget."

That's when I blurted out, "I'll never forget anything we did."

She looked at me and I think at that moment, she realized how I felt about her. I think at that moment, she realized I wasn't just the neighbor boy she became friends with but instead that I was head over heels for her. Her expression took on something akin to wonder and then sweetness. "In that case," she said, "how about a picnic?"

She could have suggested we just sit silently for twenty-four hours and I would have agreed, of course, but a picnic sounded wonderful to me. She prepared it and arrived with a basket.

We walked slowly along the shore and she eventually spread out a blanket and set up the meal. When it was ready, she sat beside me and said, "I'm really going to miss you, Andy."

I wanted to tell her that I would miss her, too, but that's when she kissed me!

It was my first ever kiss. It was the most beautiful experience of my life, and I can tell you that I don't remember anything else about the picnic at all. Afterward, we walked back, and at the door of my cabin, she kissed me one more time.

I think I floated into the house.

When I woke up in the morning, Evelyn and her parents were already gone and on their way home to Maryland. As for me, I had a full heart and a broken heart all at the same time. I didn't know how I would make it through the day, much less the years ahead.

I was in love!

The girl I loved kissed me!

And then she was gone.

I guess heartbreak always hurts but it sure felt to me like my world ended.

It didn't end, of course, and when I got home, life went on pretty much as it always had except now I had memories. In the beginning, everything made me sad. Banana splits, Joan Baez, fishing—all of the things I loved to do with her made me sad just because I wasn't doing them with her anymore. A funny thing happened, though. Eventually, the memories lost the pain and were just good memories.

It was in the middle of the first semester of my freshman year that I noticed the girl who sat next to me hummed a song I knew. It was a song I heard a lot on the shores of the lake. Noticing that made me notice she was a very pretty girl. I guess my time with Evelyn changed me because it only took me two days of thinking about Amelia before I asked her if she wanted to get ice cream after school.

We went to the shop and she ordered a hot fudge sundae. I was, of course, planning to order a banana split. Instead, I ordered a hot fudge sundae, too.

Hot fudge sundaes became my favorite.

Amelia loved the Beatles, so they replaced Joan Baez, too.

The rest of that year with Amelia was breathtaking. When the time came to go back to Lake Eerie for the summer, I didn't want to go! Amelia was going to California for the summer anyway, so we would be apart no matter what.

I didn't fall in love with Evelyn again over the summer. There was another girl, a girl in California, who had all my attention. Evelyn was busy with a boy her age anyway. I often tease Amelia that my first kiss came from someone else. She always responds that she's the one who wears my ring. She's worn my ring for closing in of fifty years now.

Action Heroes

I broke my leg when my best friend and I pretended to be action heroes and I got distracted when I noticed the girls who lived across the street were watching us. It was the summer of '87 and we had just discovered that girls weren't so bad after all. My best friend Alex and I were always coming up with crazy ideas to pass the time during the hot summer days, but today we decided to take things to a new level.

We both loved watching action movies and dreamed of being movie stars one day. So, we thought why not practice our skills and impress the girls at the same time? We grabbed some old masks and capes from our dress-up box and headed outside, ready to show off our best moves.

As we jumped and twirled around in our makeshift costumes, we could see the girls giggling and pointing in our direction. We felt like superheroes, and for a moment, nothing else mattered. That was until I pretended to fly by jumping from a tall branch, landed wrong on my leg, and heard a sickening crack.

The really crazy thing was there seemed to be a period where time just stopped. I heard the crack. Then things just stopped. There was nothing at all for a while, just silence and the knowledge that something was wrong, something hadn't turned out how I expected it to turn out. I guess now, when I think about it, I was in shock or something. At the time, it just felt like I jumped out of the tree when things were normal but when I landed, I was in some sort of confusing dream.

And then time started back up again. I remember screaming out in pain as my leg twisted beneath me, and Alex running over to help. The girls had quickly disappeared, but it didn't matter; I knew I was in trouble. I was an active boy and I'd gone through my share of scrapes and bumps but nothing could compare to the agony I felt at that moment.

What made things worse was that any movement I made seemed to affect my leg and add even more pain to the mix.

I felt weak and nauseas, and I was glad those girls couldn't see me!

Well, I went to the hospital and for a week or so, I was the hero of the neighborhood. Even the girls came by to see how I was doing. They signed my cast and flirted the way kids our age flirted. I wouldn't say it was worth the pain involved but now that pain was a dull ache instead of agony, it was hard to keep it in the front of my mind. I only had enough room there for the girls across the street and the friends who came by to sign my cast.

Well, that lasted a week or so.

And then, the fact that I couldn't do much became far more important. The rest of that summer was spent in a cast, watching as Alex and the girls played outside without me. I felt left out and alone, wondering if things would ever get better. It wasn't until one day when my dad came home with an old guitar that everything changed.

My dad played guitar back in his younger days and had always talked about teaching me. But, with all our latest adventures, we never found the time. Now that I was stuck at home, he figured it was the perfect opportunity to start. At first, I was hesitant. I didn't know anything about music, let alone playing an instrument. It didn't matter. My dad was patient and encouraging, and soon, I found myself hooked. I spent hours every day learning chords and strumming patterns, and for the first time in months, I felt like I was actually doing something. For the first time in a long time, I didn't really wonder what Alex was doing or what the girls were doing. I was lost in the excitement of the music and actually making it.

I'll never forget the day I played my first song in front of Alex, who had stopped by to check on me. It wasn't perfect, but it was a start. Alex's eyes widened in surprise, and he complimented me on my playing.

From that moment on, things started to change. I spent less time feeling sorry for myself and more time focusing on my passion. I started writing my own songs and the next year in junior high, started a band with kids from my school. I had found my place in the world, and it was on stage, playing my guitar and singing my heart out.

Man, we were horrible!

We sounded exactly like you might imagine a group of kids who could barely play sounded like. It didn't matter. We were heroes to our peers and we dreamed about being stars someday. We watched music videos on television to learn tips on performing. We played in our garages with the doors open so kids in the neighborhood would notice and drop by. In that way, we gained a small following. People would come up to us after a garage show, telling us how much they enjoyed our music. It was an incredible feeling, and I loved it.

And let me tell you, being an action hero is nothing when it comes to impressing girls! With a guitar in my hands, I was a regular heartthrob! As I grew more confident in my skills, though, a love for music became more important to me than becoming famous and having fans lined up to meet me. It even became more important than girls. In fact, by the time I was a teenager, I found myself thinking of girls as a distraction. Now, there's something you don't hear every day!

I never got famous. The truth was, I just wasn't star material. I didn't have whatever it is that stars have that puts them on the charts or sells out arenas. I became a good musician, though, and by the time I was good, I didn't really care about the rest of it. I cared about the music. I began to realize that my injury had been a blessing in disguise. Without breaking my leg, I might have never discovered my love for music. I might have continued to chase after the girls across the street, trying to impress them with my silly stunts. But instead, I had found something that truly made me happy.

The '80s were a time of change and growth. It was a decade of big hair, neon colors, and new technologies. And for me, it was a time of self-discovery. I learned that sometimes, things don't go as planned, but it's during those times that we find the most unexpected treasures of all. I kept it up with the music and even majored in music in college. I never became famous but chances are you've heard my music because I wrote a number of big songs and as a session musician, I played on a lot of albums. There are a lot of people out there who don't know my name but still know me because they sing along or bang their heads to things I created.

Years later, when I look back at that summer of '87, I smile. That was the summer I broke my leg. It was also the summer I took my very steps into what would become my life. I know it sounds crazy but I'll always be grateful for over-the-top action movies. Without them, I never would have done something stupid enough to make me discover my passion.

Fabric, Thread, and Patterns

Grandma's house was the hub of three generations of family members so it was always chaotic but the one thing that always remained perfectly organized and calm was her sewing room. It was my refuge. Whenever I needed a break from the hectic pace of life, I would go there to sit with her in her sewing room. It was not just the orderliness of the room that drew me there, but also the magical sound of the sewing machine that played like music to my ears.

The house was two stories tall but my grandfather had converted the basement for Nana. Half of the basement was pretty typical with a washing machine, a chest freezer, and a concrete floor. The other half, though, the half inside the room he constructed was pure magic. One wall had floor to ceiling shelves with fabric and spool after spool of thread in every color imaginable. There were two filing cabinets filled with patterns, two small tables, and, of course, the sewing machine. Grampa also built an island counter in the middle with a pole so she could use hangers to organize all of her works in progress.

Grandma was an excellent seamstress, and my fondest memories are of sitting on the countertop as she measured and cut fabric for one of her creations. Grandma made almost all of our clothes growing up, and I would often request specific designs. She would patiently listen to my wants and create custom dresses, skirts, or blouses. When I was in that room with her, it was like the rest of the world didn't exist at all. The rest of the world could be as loud as it wanted. In that room, everything was quiet and safe.

It was the late 1960s, and everything felt like a revolution. The cultural shift, the feminist movement, the civil rights movement, and the Vietnam War had caused significant disruptions in society. It was also the era of flower power, where hippies and young people rejected the traditional values of their parents and celebrated love, peace, and freedom.

There were many who didn't believe it was possible to make a difference, and that was on both sides of the cultural divide. The world was too big, too connected and too complicated, they would say. But within our tiny family bubble, anything seemed possible, and Grandma's needle and thread were at the center of it all. Grandma taught me in that room that I didn't have to change the world. I just had to live in it.

One day I had an idea. I wanted to make a patchwork quilt, pieced together from my old clothes that grandma had made. It was my way of keeping those clothes and the memories associated with them close. We spent hours on that quilt, cutting, piecing, trimming, and stitching. Each square told a story, and we both knew which dress, skirt or blouse it came from. Grandma shared stories of the fabrics she had used and the weather when she had made each garment. Listening to her speak about her process and share her memories was so moving. We laughed, we cried and made a beautiful quilt that I cherish to this day.

After we finished our quilt, I asked grandma to teach me to sew. She guided my hands as I stepped on the pedal of the machine, learning how to sew a straight line and make a seam. I practiced for hours, each passing moment improving my skill. Hours turned to days, and soon I was able to sew an entire blouse by myself. I was so proud of my newfound skill, and it was all thanks to Grandma's patience and guidance.

As I became more confident in my sewing abilities, I began to experiment with different types of fabrics and patterns. I discovered that, for me at least, sewing was not just a hobby but a form of expression. It allowed me to create unique and individual pieces that reflected my personal style.

It wasn't just about fashion or utilitarian purposes; sewing was also a form of activism. This was the height of the civil rights movement, and I felt empowered knowing that I could create clothing that bucked the status quo. I started making pieces that subtly promoted peace, love, and freedom. In many ways, my sewing became my way of joining the revolution.

As I honed my craft, others started to take notice. Friends and family members would often ask me to make them clothes, and I even began doing some small-scale business with local shops. With each new piece, I gained more confidence and a deeper appreciation for the power of creativity.

Years passed, and I went to college, got married, and had children of my own. But no matter where life took me, sewing remained a constant. Whenever I needed a moment of peace or a creative outlet, I turned to my trusty sewing machine.

Now, as I look back on my life, it's apparent to me that the sewing room in Grandma's house represented something much more significant than just a place to stitch fabric together. It was a refuge, a sanctuary, a creative space that allowed us to connect with one another and manifest our passions into something tangible.

The late 60s were so full of change and turmoil, but sitting in that room with grandma, surrounded by the gentle hum of sewing machines, I felt safe and secure, like everything was going to be okay. And that's the beauty of creativity, isn't it? It allows us to channel our emotions and create something meaningful, something that has the power to transcend time and connect us to the past. And, you know what? Everything became okay.

Turmoil gave way to calm and then turmoil again and then calm again and on and on because that's life. The world changed constantly and change kept up the cycle of turmoil and calm.

That wasn't just the world. That's life, too, isn't it? It was certainly true for my life. Like anyone, I had ups and downs. I had periods of chaos and periods when everything seemed organized and running smoothly. I had turmoil, and I was calm.

Through it all, I had sewing. I had grandma's sewing room and then I had one of my own. As I sit here now, surrounded by my own collection of sewing supplies, I'm reminded of the lessons I learned in Grandma's room surrounded by her supplies. I'm reminded of the patience, passion, and persistence required to create something truly unique. I'm reminded most importantly, of the joy and peace of mind it brought to my life and everyone touched by Grandma's creations and, I guess, mine as well.

See, that's why I think of sewing as art sometimes, as a creative outlet that can really make a difference. It made a difference in my life, and the truth is, it still does.

I'm afraid I have to go now. There's a teenager here. She just said, "Grandma, can you help me make a dress?"

Yes. I can help her make a dress. I most certainly can.

A Man of Respect

I stopped being ashamed of my father the day the mayor came to our tiny little shack of a house to ask my dad for advice. It was a hot summer day in 1963, and I remember wiping the sweat off my face with the sleeve of my shirt as the mayor stepped inside.

My father, a quiet man who never spoke much, seemed neither surprised nor intimidated by the sudden visit. He straightened up from where he was sitting on the porch swing and welcomed the mayor into our home. Frankly, I couldn't understand why he felt no shame about inviting the mayor, an important man, into our sparse and very humble house. I felt immediately uncomfortable. The mayor belonged in comfortable surroundings, in fancy surroundings. He didn't belong in a poor man's house.

That's what we were, poor.

So, I didn't understand why the mayor would come to our house. We had no money, and we didn't have much to offer ourselves, much less anyone else. As I listened in on their conversation, though, I realized that my father was more than just a simple carpenter.

He was a wise man.

I was eleven years old and I just never noticed that the visitors who came regularly to our house came to seek his advice. Perhaps I didn't know who they were. I knew the mayor because he'd been introduced at a school assembly and he spoke about citizenship and civic responsibility. Perhaps before that, I was just too young to understand there was a difference between people who lived in homes like ours and people who lived in large, nicer homes with beautiful yards and well-kept streets.

The mayor came to ask for my father's opinion on a new city project.

They talked for hours, discussing the details and weighing in on the pros and cons. And when the mayor left, he shook my father's hand and thanked him sincerely for his time. I didn't really understand much of the conversation. I didn't know anything about engineering or water flow or populace responses. Actually, at that point in my life, I didn't really know anything about anything at all, I suppose.

Watching my father that day changed my perspective on him, though. There was more to him than I knew. There was something others saw and others knew that I didn't. I paid attention over the next few months to those who came to see him.

A lot of people came to see him.

There came men asking about technical things, carpentry, and I guess I expected that. In addition to the mayor, there was a young man just back from college who came to him to ask his opinion about a job he was offered in the city. His father told him to talk to my father. He talked to my father about it and my father recommended against taking it. It was another conversation I didn't fully understand but six months later, there was a scandal at that company and a number of employees were arrested.

I couldn't understand how my father was so regularly sought after. He was just a poor worker! Our town wasn't large but it seemed large enough to me that my father was just one of many faces of poor folks in the valley instead of rich folks in the hills.

He wasn't, though. Over the months that followed, I paid attention, I realized that he was a man of substance, someone who had earned the respect of others despite his humble circumstances. It inspired me to look at myself differently too, to see that I could achieve great things if I worked hard enough and believed in myself. I never asked him about the respect others showed him. I never tried to figure out what might have brought him to that point. I just set out trying to be a man of respect.

Since the only respected man I knew was my father, I set out trying to be like him.

I accompanied him to his job as often as I could and I would hold his tools or help him measure. I learned carpentry from a master and though I didn't really learn what made people respect him, by the time I was fifteen, I wasn't just holding his tools. I worked alongside him and I even had my own paycheck. The summer I turned sixteen, I felt like the world was changing fast. There were civil rights movements and protests happening all around us. There were war protestors and war supporters. There were new ideas about cosmic consciousness, the Age of Aquarius, and expanding your mind.

My father was still my father, quietly going about his work as he always had.

While the world around us seemed tumultuous, my father seemed as serene as he always had. He went about his days with the same quiet strength he always had. One day as we drove home from a construction site, I asked him about all the protests and all the chaos in the world. I asked him what he thought about it, if he agreed with the protestors.

"I'm starting a new project," he said. "I'm building a community hall where people can come together and share ideas. And I want you to help me."

That was his response. He was building something and wanted my help.

I didn't know how to respond. I suppose to an extent I thought this was some kind of coded lesson, like he was somehow giving me a message of wisdom I needed to work out. On the other hand, I also thought he might just be avoiding the question the way a number of people tried to avoid political conversations all together. I didn't know. What I knew, though, was that helping him work was something I loved so I readily agreed.

Over the next few months, we worked tirelessly on the community hall. My father taught me more about carpentry, and we spent long hours measuring, sawing, and hammering away. It was hard work, but it was satisfying too. It was the first time I really paid attention to the results, the first time I noticed clearly that something tangible emerged from our labor, something that would benefit the people in our community.

As the project progressed, volunteers showed up to help. It was only then that I learned this project was something my father did for free. He got the town to pay for supplies but he didn't take a single red cent for himself. When I learned that, I set aside the money he gave me every week and put it in a shoebox under my bed.

We worked on the hall day and night. It was exhausting but it was also exhilarating, knowing that I was building something that would last long after I was gone. It felt different than the houses I'd help build or even the playground. It felt special and the way others joined in felt special as well. Finally, the day came when we opened the doors of the community hall. People from town and from the surrounding towns showed up, eager to see what we had built.

It was not just a building, it was a symbol of hope, a place where people could come together and work towards a better future. My father gave a speech, thanking everyone who had helped with the project, and I stood next to him, beaming with pride.

And then I understood.

My father was respected because he cared.

He told me time and time again over the years, "People don't care how much you know until they know how much you care." I never understood that. It was just one of those sayings I supposed all parents told their children. Right then, though, I knew what it meant. I understood. My father was respected because people could trust any advice he gave was given with no ulterior motives, no selfish desires, and nothing but the best intentions for the people involved.

Now, over fifty years later, that community hall still stands, a testament to the hard work and determination of a group of people led by a man determined to build it. I return to my hometown from time to time with my daughter and her family. I always get her to drive us by the community center and every time we do, I feel a sense of pride and accomplishment, knowing that I played a small part in its creation. I feel a great deal more pride for my father, knowing the part he played was the one part absolutely necessary.

Because he was a man worthy of respect.

Groupie

My first concert happened when I was eighteen years old. I went with a group of friends to see a band who wasn't famous and whose music I didn't even know. I still ended up being a groupie even though I didn't even like their music. It was the 1970s, and I was just a young girl trying to find my place in the world, I suppose. I was caught up in the excitement of being with rock stars.

Well, they weren't rock stars but they behaved like they were.

Alcohol, drugs, plenty of sex.

I was eighteen years old and I had my experience with all of those things, growing up in an era when those things were taken lightly by youth and all but tolerated by society.

I had always been drawn to music and the freedom it seemed to provide. So, when my friends said to go see the band playing at a local venue, I couldn't resist the allure of seeing rock and roll live and in person for the first time in my life. As I entered the little warehouse converted into a concert hall, I could feel the energy buzzing around me. Young people just like me laughed and danced together, all united by this universal language of music.

I found myself swept up in the excitement, and before I knew it, I was dancing with a group of people I had never met before. It was liberating to forget about all of my worries and just enjoy the moment. We danced to two opening acts who were, frankly, much better than the headliners.

On the other hand, when the main event happened, I noticed that the lead singer was very cute, the guitarists was bad-boy attractive, and the drummer was probably the best-looking human being who had ever walked the face of the earth.

The band wasn't very good, but I didn't mind. They were good looking and their passion for music and the way they connected with the crowd was infectious. I found myself wanting to learn more about them and their world. So, after the show, I went backstage to meet the band. They were just a group of regular guys, but they had something special. They welcomed me with open arms and treated me like I was part of their group.

There were five band members, and three other girls like me back there. We talked and drank and when the girls started kissing the guys, I joined in, too. We all ended up in their converted school bus and I just traveled with them to their next gig. I traveled with them for the whole summer, a girlfriend (one of four) for the whole band. It was crazy. It was unwise. It was an immature and silly thing to do.

It was the best experience of my life.

It wasn't about the music or the fame. It wasn't about the sex and drugs and rock and roll. It wasn't even about being on the road or living a life that felt free of responsibility or worry. It was about connection and adventure. It was about, I guess, the idea of love expressed abundantly and freely. None of the band members expected to ever be famous. They were just good enough to get booked in little venues or at bars for a share of the booze receipts.

We went from place to place, a summer of constant exploration. I got to see it through the lenses of different perspectives, too, because in one place, I might be with the drummer but in the next, I'd be with the bass player. The lead singer and I went to a zoo and there was something magical about that. I learned so much about myself and the world around me. I wasn't thinking about my future. I wasn't thinking about my past. I was thinking about the moment.

Right now.

Right this very instant.

I always thought that music was a powerful tool that could heal wounds and bring people together. It could inspire us, make us feel alive, and give us hope for a better future. I thought that was probably true but for me, the music was just an excuse for all of the rest to follow. Through my experiences with the band, I grew in ways that I never could have imagined. I became more confident and independent, and I learned to appreciate the beauty in simple things.

We lost two of the other groupies along the way. One got possessive of the guitar player and ended up with a bus ticket back home. Another just got tired. The constant party became too much for her. We picked up another girl, though, and Tami and I became close friends. I was grateful for that first concert and the experiences that followed. It opened up countless possibilities for me and helped me find my place in the world.

We finished our summer circuit. The route was arranged in a circle and so the very last show was right back where we started. I spent a final night at the motel with the lead singer and then kissed him goodbye. The tour was over and so were my days as a groupie. In the end, it wasn't about the band or the music, but it was about the journey and the connections I made along the way.

That's what makes life worth living, right? It's all about experiencing new things, meeting new people, and creating memories that last a lifetime.

Tami got off the bus in my hometown and stayed at my house for a month before we got an apartment together. We both went to community college and then transferred to the state university. A few years after college, I started a family of my own. A few years later, Tami did as well. The lessons I learned during those days have never left me. They have become a part of who I am and have shaped the way I see the world.

Tami and I are still close and every now and then we go online to see if there's anything about the band. So far, we can't find a single mention on the internet.

Of course, we still have recordings of the shows, and every now and then, we'll get together and laugh as we talk about that summer. Our grandchildren always look at us in wonder, two old ladies who lived a crazy, wild life.

Maybe were a little wild.

Maybe we were a little crazy.

But I don't think we actually started living life until after that summer.

Shoulder Pads

All my friends made fun of the silly poofy shoulders in women's business fashion, and I made fun of those shoulders, too, even though my sixteen-year-old sense of taste actually found them quite alluring. I was an awkward teenager, with big glasses and braces, and more interested in books than fashion. When I was interested in fashion, it was always from an intellectual standpoint. Shoulder pads were functional necessities with some fabrics because of the weight of the cloth. That was a fact I understood. Shoulder pads a choice started as an attempt to emulate Japanese traditional wear with the shoulders extended to make the waist look smaller. That was another fact. That was something easy to process.

But my life was about to change drastically, in a way that would make me realize that fashion was the least of my worries. It all started when my family moved from the city to a small town in the countryside. My parents wanted a quieter, more affordable life, and they figured the best place to find it was in a tiny house on a farm outside of town. I was hesitant at first, leaving all my friends behind, but I soon discovered that there was something special about this new life.

I made friends with the animals on the farm, especially a horse named Sparrow who became my best friend. I learned how to ride, how to milk cows, how to grow vegetables, and how to fix things around the house. I also joined a new school, where I quickly realized that I was the odd one out. Most of the students had grown up in the area, and they were all into different things than I was. They listened to country music, wore cowboy boots and hats, and talked about hunting and fishing. I felt like an outsider, but I didn't let that stop me.

One day, I saw a flyer on the bulletin board for a local talent show. It was the kind of thing I had never done before, but I felt like I needed to try something new.

I decided to write a poem, something that expressed my feelings about the farm and the animals. I would write the poem and then perform it in front of the whole school.

I practiced every day, reciting my lines to Sparrow and the cows. They seemed to enjoy it, or at least they didn't run away. I got nervous as the day of the talent show approached, but I kept telling myself that it didn't matter if I made a fool of myself. What mattered was that I was doing something that scared me.

On the day of the show, I put on my best outfit (which wasn't saying much) and went to school with butterflies in my stomach. When it was my turn to go on stage, I felt like running away. But I didn't. I walked up there, took a deep breath, and said my poem.

It wasn't perfect. I stumbled on a few words, I spoke too fast in some parts and too slow in others. But when I finished, the room was silent. Then, slowly, people started clapping, and before I knew it, the whole auditorium was filled with applause. I had never felt so proud of myself in my life.

I don't think my poem was very good.

I don't think I performed it very well.

The applause wasn't for the performance. Everyone was shocked and impressed that I had the guts to do something like that, that I was willing to get up there and share something that wasn't, like poofy shoulders, already popular and accepted.

After that day, things changed for me. Kids at school started talking to me more, asking about my life before the new town and also about my life on the farm. They invited me to go fishing and I went. They invited me to go hunting with them and I went. I didn't become one of them overnight, but I no longer felt like an outsider.

And then, a few weeks later, something happened that would change everything once again. A new girl arrived at school. Her name was Sarah, and she was unlike anyone I had ever met before. She had short hair. She wore leather jackets and ripped jeans and listened to punk rock music. She didn't seem to care what anyone thought of her, and that made her fascinating to me.

I had to work up the courage to do that poem! It seemed like she would never have felt nervous in the first place.

I approached her one day during lunchtime, deciding to take a risk. "Hey, I'm Mary," I said. "Would you like to sit with me?"

To my surprise, she smiled and told me she'd love to. Sarah and I ate together and talked about music and books, and soon we had discovered that we had a lot in common. She told me about how she had been bullied in her old school for being different but it just made her rebel against conformity more. As we walked home together that day, talking and laughing, we joked about shoulder pads and poofy shoulders.

She came to the farm and she stared in wonder at the animals. She insisted on helping me gather eggs and she got her first taste of fresh eggs when Mom scrambled dome for us. It felt like we were instant best friends, and we made a pact to always be ourselves even if that meant being different from everyone around us.

And so, in the fall of 1986, I went to the thrift store and bought myself a leather jacket, a pair of boots, and a tee shirt with a punk rock band on it. I wore them proudly, even with my big glasses and braces, and nobody laughed at me. Sarah became my closest friend, and we spent hours listening to punk rock and talking about our dreams, our fears, and our hopes for the future.

Years later, when I look back on that time in my life, I realize that it was a turning point for me.

It was when I learned to chase my own happiness, regardless of what everyone else thought. And it was when I met the people who would inspire me to become who I am today.

It's crazy to think my first thoughts on all this came because of shoulder pads.

All because of some silly poofy shoulders in women's business fashion that we all made fun of.

Now, when I see fashion trends come and go, I remember that lesson. It's not about fitting in or being conventional. It's about being true to who you are, expressing yourself, and finding your own path in life. And I know that wherever I go, whatever I do, I'll always be thankful for that time in the decade of excess when I learned to be myself.

Think I'm Just Happy

By the time I turned thirty-four, I'd switched from the heavy metal music I loved growing up to the new sound from the Seattle scene, grunge music. It was like a breath of fresh air for me. The rawness and authenticity spoke to my soul in a way that metal never could. I had always felt like an outsider, but listening to grunge made me feel like I had found a community of like-minded outsiders, outsiders who were inside after all.

It was in 1991 that the whole world felt the power of grunge. People couldn't even understand what Curt Cobain sang but they sang along, nonetheless. As for me, the music was unlike anything I had ever heard before. I was immediately hooked. I spent hours listening to grunge music and reading articles about in music magazines.

But the year also brought some personal challenges for me. I was going through a divorce and trying to navigate life as a single parent to my two young children. It was a difficult time, but the music provided me with a sense of comfort and escapism. And, I guess, I ought to admit there was something amazing and fun about a five-year-old boy and a six-year-old girl singing about the smell of teen spirit. There were moments of joy in the midst of the pain but the pain sometimes seemed far, far more overwhelming than the joy felt good.

I was salesman and at that moment, I needed a salesperson to provide me with a solution, to overcome my objections, and to close the deal. I needed someone to show up to sell me a big box of happiness. Of course, nobody showed up at my front door carrying a box like that.

One day, while I was listening to another band talking about a homeless man resting his head on a pillow made of concrete, I realized if I was going to buy a box of happiness, I would have to be the one to sell it to myself. I couldn't change that my wife left me.

I couldn't change that she abandoned the kids. I couldn't change any of that but that didn't mean there was nothing I could do.

I decided that I needed to do something to change my life for the better. I couldn't continue living with sadness and negativity as my primary emotions and with my music being the only thing that let me get through it all. My kids deserved a father more engaged with this life. They deserved a father who could teach them to live energetically and enthusiastically.

So, I made a list of things that I wanted to accomplish and set out to achieve them.

My first goal was to get a new job. I had been working in sales for years, but it wasn't fulfilling me anymore. I made the money we needed. In fact, finances was the one area of my life I'd somehow managed to always keep under control.

I wanted to do something more meaningful with my life, though. So, I started looking for opportunities in the non-profit sector. After months of searching and attending job interviews, I finally landed a position as a fundraising coordinator for a regional charity. The charity provided housing and transportation for families who had to travel to other cities for medical treatment, and that was critical in the middle of the AIDs epidemic.

My next goal was to improve my physical health. I had always been overweight and lacked confidence in my appearance. I got a stationary bicycle and I stacked seven CDs next to the stereo. That was seven days a week and every day I biked to the sound of one album. The exercise was easier than the dietary changes but I fought through it. It was tough at first, but I soon noticed a difference in my energy levels and overall well-being.

As the year went on, I started to gain more confidence in myself. I was proud of the progress I had made and felt like I was finally moving in the right direction. The world was also changing. Major events were happening all around us. The Soviet Union collapsed. There was war in the Middle East. AIDs devastated whole communities. Poverty. Gang violence. It seemed like the world, just like me, had problems.

But I was working on my problems and I worked for a nonprofit that worked on some of the bigger problems. I grew stronger and happier. I don't know if my kids noticed a difference at all! To them, I was the same Daddy I'd always been. I don't think they even noticed I'd lost fifty pounds. I was still the man who sang with them, who sat down with them for dinner, and who helped them through the nights when they missed their mother and wondered why she never came back.

And so, I entered 1991 as one version of myself and entered 1992 as a version I liked much better. At thirty-four, I was unhappy, unhealthy, and inspired. At thirty-five I was confident my life could have meaning.

The kids' mother never came back. Instead, I remarried in 1993, and Leah replaced the mother they'd lost. She was like grunge music for me, replacing my wife the way the Seattle Scene replaced my old music. There was one critical difference, though. Even to this day, I'll occasionally listen to Iron Maiden or Flotsam and Jetsam, a little metal in the midst of the grunge. With my ex-wife, it's different. Like my sales job and the extra weight, she's something in my past that has no purpose in my present. My life has enough purpose now that there's no reason to muddle things up.

That year was transformative for me, and I guess that year is filled with the most powerful memories of my life.

Not the best memories.

Those memories are still to be made!

Made in the USA
Monee, IL
20 November 2023

46952014R00057